Medical Education
at a Glance

This title is also available as an e-book.
For more details, please see
www.wiley.com/buy/9781118723883
or scan this QR code:

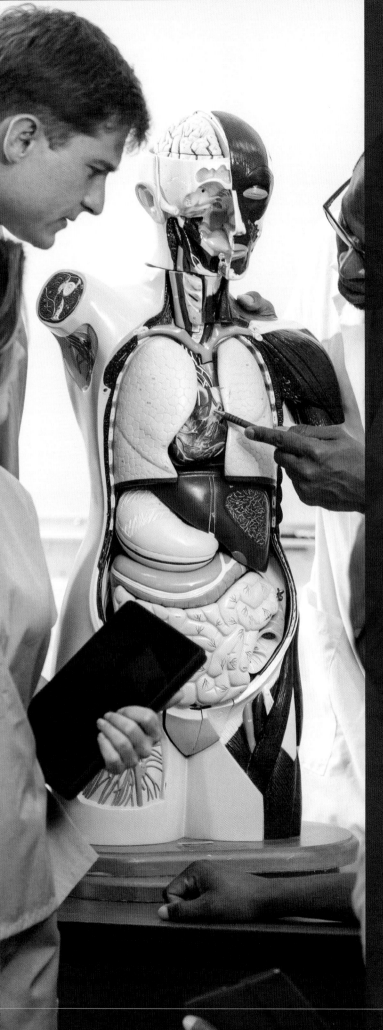

Medical Education at a Glance

Edited by
Judy McKimm
Professor of Medical Education and Director of Strategic Educational Development
Swansea University Medical School
Swansea, UK

Visiting Professor
Princess Nourah bint Abdulrahman University
Riyadh, Kingdom of Saudi Arabia

Guest Professor
Huazhong University of Science and Technology
Wuhan, China

Kirsty Forrest
Professor, Deputy Head Medicine
Faculty of Health Sciences and Medicine
Bond University, Australia

Jill Thistlethwaite
Professor, Medical Adviser
NPS MedicineWise
Sydney, Australia

Health Professional Education Consultant
and Adjunct Professor
University of Technology Sydney
Sidney, Australia

Honorary Professor
School of Education
University of Queensland, Australia

WILEY Blackwell

Registered Offices: John Wiley & Sons, Inc., 111 River Street, Hoboken, NJ 07030, USA
John Wiley & Sons Ltd, The Atrium, Southern Gate, Chichester, West Sussex, PO19 8SQ, UK

Editorial Office: 9600 Garsington Road, Oxford, OX4 2DQ, UK

For details of our global editorial offices, customer services, and more information about Wiley products visit us at www.wiley.com.

Wiley also publishes its books in a variety of electronic formats and by print-on-demand. Some content that appears in standard print versions of this book may not be available in other formats.

Limit of Liability/Disclaimer of Warranty

Library of Congress Cataloging-in-Publication Data
Names: McKimm, Judy, editor. | Forrest, Kirsty, editor. | Thistlethwaite, Jill, editor.
Title: Medical education at a glance / Judy McKimm, Kirsty Forrest, Jill Thistlethwaite.
Other titles: At a glance series (Oxford, England)
Description: First edition. | Hoboken, NJ : John Wiley & Sons, Inc., 2017. |
   Series: At a glance series | Includes bibliographical references and index.
Identifiers: LCCN 2016045903 (print) | LCCN 2016046543 (ebook) | ISBN
   9781118723883 (pbk.) | ISBN 9781118723814 (pdf) | ISBN 9781118723821 (epub)
Subjects: | MESH: Education, Medical
Classification: LCC R735 (print) | LCC R735 (ebook) | NLM W 18 | DDC
   610.71–dc23
LC record available at https://lccn.loc.gov/2016045903

Cover image: © kali9/Gettyimages

Set in 9.5/11.5 Minion Pro by Aptara, India
Printed and bound in Singapore by Markono Print Media Pte Ltd

10 9 8 7 6 5 4 3 2 1

Contents

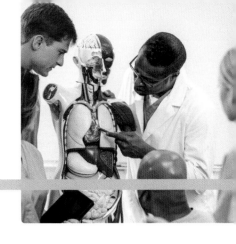

Part 1 Overview and broad concepts   1

Part 2 Medical education in practice   27

Part 3 Assessment and feedback   77

Preface

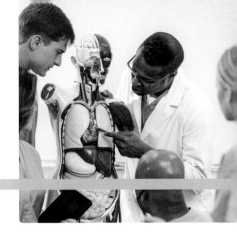

Welcome to the first edition of *Medical Education at a Glance*. This book was conceived as an introduction to key aspects of medical education, which would provide an accessible overview for those new to medical education or a handy summary for those more experienced. We also envisaged that it would provide a taster for medical educators who might then wish to explore the more substantial books produced by Wiley such as *Understanding Medical Education* (2nd edition) and *Researching Medical Education*.

Medical Education at a Glance will be relevant to doctors, dentists, nurses and other healthcare professionals at various levels (including students), as well as to support staff. The book is particularly appropriate for guiding medical students and doctors in training and their teachers, supervisors, mentors and trainers. It aims to inform and encourage those engaged in improving education and training. As well as the chapters written by ourselves, we have been fortunate in attracting additional contributors with huge expertise and knowledge about medical education in both the academic and clinical environments.

In the usual at a Glance style, the book is designed to summarise what are often fairly complex or substantial topics, so that readers learn some of the language and key terms while gaining a broad understanding of the topic. Given this approach, we cannot go into depth on any one area and so further reading and resources are identified for each topic for the reader to explore further. What we have aimed to do is provide an introduction to some key educational concepts as they relate to clinical practice and university-based education. We have tried to make the chapters practically focussed with examples of how concepts or approaches might be applied in practice. Each chapter (or group of chapters) is free standing, although reading the whole book will provide a good grounding in medical education theory and practice.

The book begins with an overview and introduction to medical education, its purpose, structure and predominant educational or learning theories. It also considers some of the core aspects of contemporary education including curriculum, selection, leadership and international contexts. We move on to consider approaches to learning and teaching planning and implementation in different contexts and with different groups of learners. The later chapters consider assessment and feedback in both the academic and clinical environments. A comprehensive further reading, resources and reference list concludes the book. We hope that you enjoy the book, and that it stimulates you to reflect on and develop your own educational practice and that of others.

Judy McKimm, Kirsty Forrest and *Jill Thistlethwaite*

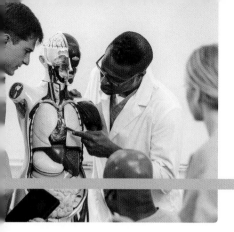

Acknowledgements

We would like to acknowledge all the contributing authors who have offered different perspectives on various aspects of medical education. The book reflects our experiences over many years working with learners, teachers and patients in a range of international contexts and we would also like to acknowledge their contribution to our understanding of medical education. Finally, as ever, we'd like to thank our partners – Andy, Derek and George – for their unfailing support and patience.

About the editors

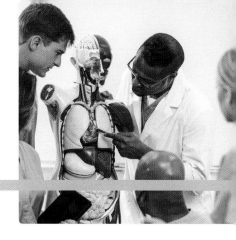

Judy McKimm

Judy's current role is Director of Strategic Educational Development and Professor of Medical Education in the College of Medicine, Swansea University. From 2011 to 2014, she was Dean of Medical Education at Swansea and before that worked in New Zealand from 2007 to 2011, at the University of Auckland and as Pro-Dean, Health and Social Care, Unitec Institute of Technology. Judy initially trained as a nurse and has an academic background in social and health sciences, education and management. She was Director of Undergraduate Medicine at Imperial College London until 2004 and led the curriculum development and implementation of a new undergraduate medical programme. In 2004–2005, as Higher Education Academy Senior Adviser, she was responsible for developing and implementing the accreditation of professional development programmes and the standards for teachers in HE. She has worked on over 60 international health workforce and education reform projects for DfID, AusAID, the World Bank and WHO in Central Asia, Portugal, Greece, Bosnia and Herzegovina, Macedonia, Australia and the Pacific. She has been a reviewer and accreditor for the GMC, QAA, the Higher Education Academy and the Academy of Medical Educators for many years and is a member of ASME Executive and Council. She is programme director for the Leadership Masters at Swansea and Director of ASME's international Educational Leadership programme. She writes and publishes widely on medical education and leadership and runs health professions' leadership and education courses and workshops internationally. Her most recent books are *Global Health* (with Brian Nicholson and Ann Allen), *Health Care Professionalism at a Glance* (with Jill Thistlethwaite), *Clinical Leadership Made Easy* (with Helen O'Sullivan) and the *ABC of Clinical Leadership,* 2nd edition (with Tim Swanwick).

Kirsty Forrest

Kirsty is Deputy Head of Medicine in the Faculty of Health Sciences and Medicine at Bond University, Australia. Prior to this she was Associate Dean, Learning and Teaching and Director of Medical Education in the Faculty of Medicine and Health Sciences Macquarie University (2013–2016). She moved from the UK where she was an Honorary Senior Lecturer at the University of Leeds (2005–2013) and Clinical Education Advisor for the Yorkshire and Humber Deanery (2009–2013). She received her medical degree from the University of Edinburgh and has specialty fellowships in anaesthesia from the UK and the Australian and New Zealand Anaesthetic Colleges, and continues to work clinically. She has a Masters in Medical Education from the University of Sheffield and has coauthored and edited a number of medical textbooks. These include: *How to Teach Continuing Medical Education, Essential Guide to Acute Care, Professional Practice for Foundation Doctors – Becoming Tomorrow's Doctors, Essential Guide to Educational Supervision in Postgraduate Medical Education* and *Simulation in Clinical Education.*

Jill Thistlethwaite

Jill Thistlethwaite is a health professional education consultant, medical adviser at NPS MedicineWise and adjunct professor at University of Technology Sydney. She received her medical degree from University College London and has since practised as a general practitioner (family doctor) in both the UK and Australia. She received her PhD on the topic of shared decision making and medical education from the University of Maastricht. For over 20 years she has worked across the continuum of health professional education at undergraduate, postgraduate and continuing professional development (CPD) levels. Her main interests are interprofessional education (IPE) and collaborative practice, professionalism and communication skills. Jill has written/coedited several books and book chapters, and has published over 90 papers in peer-reviewed journals. Her most recently published books are: *Values-based Interprofessional Collaborative Practice*; *Health Care Professionalism at a Glance* with Judy McKimm and *Leading Research and Evaluation in Interprofessional Education* coedited with Dawn Forman and Marion Jones. She is coeditor-in-chief of *The Clinical Teacher* and an associate editor of the *Journal of Interprofessional Care.* In 2014, she was a Fulbright Senior Scholar at the National Center for Interprofessional Practice and Education in the USA.

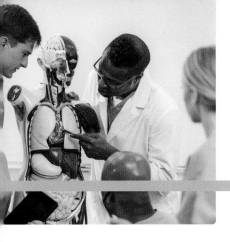

Contributors

Michelle McLean, Chapter 12
Professor of Medical Education and Academic lead for PBL, Bond University, Australia

Andrew Grant, Chapter 26
Practising GP and Professor and Dean of Medical Education, Swansea University Medical School, UK

Nicola Cooper, Chapter 27
Consultant Physician & Hon Clinical Associate Professor, Derby Teaching Hospitals NHS Foundation Trust, and Division of Medical Sciences & Graduate Entry Medicine, University of Nottingham, UK

Claire Vogan, Chapter 32
Associate Professor and Director of Student Support and Guidance, Swansea University Medical School, UK

Sean Smith, Chapter 35
Systems Developer, Bradford Institute for Health Research, Bradford Teaching Hospitals NHS Trust, UK

Sam May, Chapter 36
Lecturer in Medical Education, Swansea University Medical School, UK

Heidi Phillips, Chapter 37
Practising GP and Admissions Director for Graduate Entry Medical Programme, Swansea University Medical School, UK

Luci Etheridge, Chapters 38–41, 44
Consultant Paediatrician, St George's University Healthcare NHS Foundation Trust, and Honorary Senior Lecturer, St George's, University of London, UK

Rebecca Hodgkinson, Paediatric Registrar at Evelina London Children's Hospital, Former Chair London School of Paediatrics Trainee Committee and Former Trainee representative RCPCH Assessment Committee

Kathy Boursicot, Director, Professional Assessment Consultancy, Singapore

Overview and broad concepts

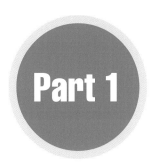

Part 1

Chapters

1 What is medical education?

Practice points

- Medical education draws from a range of disciplines to design and deliver programmes, and engage in research with a common goal of ensuring doctors are caring, competent and safe to practice
- It is jointly delivered by universities and healthcare providers
- Medical educators need to be aware of global trends and issues and challenges arising from both the education and healthcare sectors

Table 1.1 Issues in international higher education and health care

Issues in higher education	Issues in health care
'Massification' (huge growth) of university-based education	Demand for healthcare practitioners outstripping supply
Impact of learning technologies (e.g. simulation, mobile learning)	Impact of technologies (e.g. remote monitoring of conditions, telemedicine)
Student/learner expectations	Patient expectations
Cost of delivery	Workforce maldistribution
Preparing for employability in a changing, global environment	Increase in non-communicable disease, pandemics, antimicrobial resistance
Internationalisation – threats from the global market	Community/primary care emphasis
Equality and diversity of staff and students, including unequal access and outcomes	Inequalities of health access and outcome within and between countries
Regulation and quality control of education	Environmental threats

Figure 1.1 Medical education: a global movement

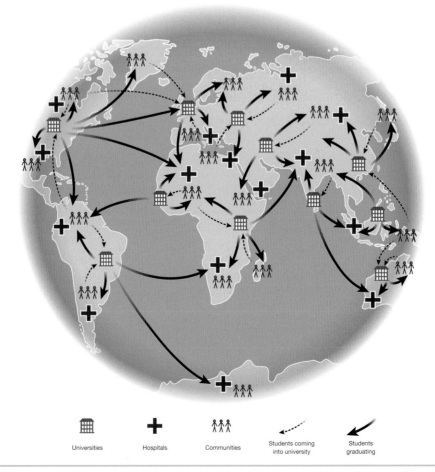

Medical Education at a Glance, First Edition. Edited by Judy McKimm, Kirsty Forrest and Jill Thistlethwaite © 2017 John Wiley & Sons, Ltd. Published 2017 by John Wiley & Sons, Ltd.

Medical education is 'the process of teaching, learning and training of students with an ongoing integration of knowledge, experience, skills, qualities, responsibility and values which qualify an individual to practice medicine. It is divided into undergraduate, postgraduate and continuing medical education, but increasingly there is a focus on the "lifelong" nature of medical education.' (IIME, 2016).

Medical education has evolved over the last century to become a discrete educational field of study, which has shaped not only the way doctors are educated and trained but has also influenced wider education. Prior to the Flexner Report (Flexner, 1910), medical education was undertaken on an apprenticeship model, and it was usually the most privileged and wealthy who had access to such training. The Flexner Report recommended that the American and Canadian medical school system be transformed to one which provided university education in the basic medical sciences and also trained students in the workplace to be practising clinicians. Since then, around the world, basic (undergraduate or prequalifying) medical education has moved into universities, and medical education at all stages has become ever more tightly controlled and regulated.

Professionals who are involved in the education of students, doctors in training and qualified practitioners are termed medical educators. Medical educators come from a range of backgrounds: education, other health professions and the social and behavioural sciences, as well as from the biomedical sciences and medical specialties (i.e. practising clinicians). Doctors' world views and paradigms have traditionally reflected positivism, the scientific method and the pragmatism of the *real world*. This is both a strength and a weakness: a strength in that it can bring scientific rigour to research, and engagement in everyday clinical practice brings authenticity to teaching, learning and practice-based research; a weakness in that 'medical education is about people and the way we think, act and interact in the world. Medical education research is not a poor relation of medical research; it belongs to a different family altogether' (Monrouxe and Rees, 2009, p. 198).

Currently, a range of approaches in medical education practice and research exists – from social, behavioural and management sciences, and the humanities as well as from more traditional disciplines. This has led to a richness and diversity of activities and outcomes, which utilise different approaches from other subject disciplines (particularly school and adult education) to explore what works, why and how? in the real world. For example, situational, experiential and outcomes-based education are derived from general education; and patient safety and simulation education was extended and adapted from work done in the airline and nuclear industry. And the 'taken for granted' role of reflection in developing medical professionals drew heavily on Schön's (a philosopher) work on learning organisations and the reflective practitioner (e.g. Schön, 1987). See later chapters.

Medical education also gives back to the wider education and health community through specific educational strategies and social accountability initiatives: the social good of Tan *et al.* (2011). For example, problem-based learning (PBL), developed at McMaster University, Canada in the 1960s, is now used in many educational sectors and the objective structured clinical examination or OSCE (Harden and Gleeson, 1979) is now widely used in veterinary and health professions' education.

Professional education and training

The first professions established were medicine, divinity and law, and medical doctors continue to have a very privileged position in society. It is partly because of the high status of medicine that medical education is somewhat set apart from the education and training of other health professionals. Medical schools often operate semi-autonomously, have relatively high power, utilise different funding streams and offer higher rates of remuneration for their clinical teachers than other disciplines (Swanwick, 2014). At postgraduate level, doctors have one of the longest training periods of any professional before they are deemed fit for independent practice, typically overseen by specially established postgraduate colleges.

Despite these differences, medical schools have to abide by the rules and regulations of the universities in which they reside in order to be able to award medical degrees. Programme approval and quality assurance mechanisms operate in exactly the same way for medical programmes as they do for any other programme. Medical education and training (and the activities of individual doctors) is subject to regulation from regulatory and professional bodies (e.g. medical councils), just as other health and social care professions are. Basic medical education and training (just as in undergraduate nursing, social work or physiotherapy programmes) is delivered both in the workplace and the university, with the involvement of practitioners and others not directly employed by the university.

Current concerns and issues

Many of the concerns in medical education are those experienced by all higher education and health organisations (Table 1.1). Medical education needs to take account not only of educational concerns and issues, but also those affecting the health services in which the training and education are carried out. At the heart of medical education is the need to produce and maintain safe, competent, caring doctors, so patient safety and fitness to practice issues are high on the agenda. Simulation and the use of computer-based and mobile learning technologies are helping to prepare learners for clinical practice, although they can never compensate for learning from real patients, their families and communities. Changes in health structures and systems, the impact of technologies resulting in shorter inpatients' stays and consequent limitations on clinical placements have huge impact on the type and quality of clinical education that can be provided.

Both health care and education are now global industries and, in many countries the numbers of student places in programmes are capped. Due to these factors, as well as universities becoming more entrepreneurial, many medical schools are seeking other ways (including developing collaborations with overseas partners) to expand student numbers. The expanding knowledge base in medicine and consequent curriculum pressures are leading educators to explore different curricular models as they prepare students and doctors for 21st century practice (Lueddeke, 2012) (see Chapter 6). The internationalisation of medical educators is reflected in the way individuals, groups and organisations collaborate and share practice and ideas around the world. Whilst this rich diversity of perspectives may lead to debate and disagreement about the *right* way to do things, all medical educators share a common purpose: to provide medical education that leads to those who engage in it striving to provide the best health care to the patients and communities they serve.

2 Stages of medical education

Practice points

Broadly, four distinct stages exist in medical education and training:
- Basic medical education – delivered by universities in collaboration with health providers
- Early postgraduate or internship, where the newly qualified doctor works under close supervision
- Specialist postgraduate training, where the doctor trains for a particular specialty or career
- Continuing professional development and updating

Table 2.1   The four stages of medical education

Stage	Who is involved	Key features	Years (approx.)
Basic medical education	Medical students	This is a university-based 'medical degree' Students enter after secondary school (undergraduates) or after another degree (graduate entry)	4–7
Early postgraduate	Doctors in training e.g. Junior Doctor, Foundation Doctor, Intern	Early career doctors, retain generalist roles Under direct supervision Geared towards achieving defined competencies	1–2
Postgraduate specialty	Doctors in training, e.g. Resident, Registrar	Training for a particular specialty/career, e.g. a 'surgeon' or a 'psychiatrist' and/or on academic/ teaching/research pathways Working under supervision to a defined curriculum and competencies Involved in training juniors and students	4+
Continuing Professional Development (CPD) Continuing Medical Education (CME)	All practising, registered doctors	Maintaining, updating, diversifying, subspecialising Often linked to formal appraisal, relicensing and revalidating processes	Ongoing – the rest of your career

Source: adapted from McKimm *et al.,* 2013.

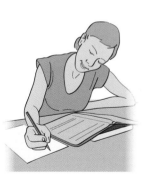
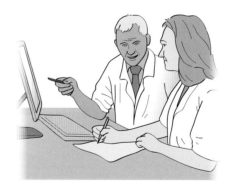
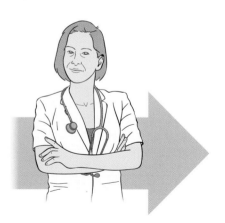

The stages of medical education comprise basic (undergraduate) medical education, postgraduate medical education (including vocational training, specialist training, and research doctoral education), continuing medical education (CME) and the continuing professional development (CPD) of medical doctors (WFME, 2016).

Basic medical education

Basic or undergraduate medical education refers to the period that begins when a student enters medical school and ends with the final examination for basic medical qualification. In some countries, however, undergraduate education refers to pre-medical college education, which results in a Bachelor's degree and is the training students receive before entering medical school.

Basic medical education is usually provided by universities, whose programmes are accredited by a regulatory body (such as a medical council). Accreditation is a quality assurance process that aims to evaluate educational and training institutions, programmes and practices to determine whether applicable (i.e. national and/ or international) standards are met. Increasingly, undergraduate programme accreditation is tied to the regulation and licensing of health professionals, most commonly to initial licensing and registration.

Medical Education at a Glance, First Edition. Edited by Judy McKimm, Kirsty Forrest and Jill Thistlethwaite © 2017 John Wiley & Sons, Ltd. Published 2017 by John Wiley & Sons, Ltd.

Successful completion of medical programmes leads graduates to professional registration and entry into postgraduate training. Many programmes also include opportunities for additional full-time study leading to an intercalated degree, such as a BSc, Masters or PhD in a related science or social science.

Worldwide, two main curriculum models for basic medical education exist, although within these a variety of educational offerings are provided:

1 **traditional undergraduate programme**, lasting 5–7 years, primarily for school leavers;
2 **graduate entry programmes**, lasting 4–5 years for graduates with a prior university degree or qualified health professionals. Students on these programmes are also referred to as medical students and can leave with further Bachelors', or more frequently Masters' qualifications. The Masters' degrees often include a strong element of research training.

The latter, most notably in Australia, North America and Europe, are new professional degrees based on the broad-based undergraduate degrees. The rationale behind such shifts was in response to international changes, such as the Bologna Agreement (European Commission, 2015), which aims to streamline and align all higher education programmes and levels in the EU. See Chapter 6 for further description of curriculum models.

Postgraduate training

Internationally, effective postgraduate education is highly structured with clear definition of standards, outcomes and competencies delivered by trained supervisors and measured by a wide range of assessments, as described in Chapters 38–44.

In many low and middle income countries (LMICs), however, whilst basic medical education may be offered, it is at postgraduate level, and in particular in speciality training, that more development is needed. In some areas this has been addressed at regional level through defining standards and sharing resources. Reciprocal agreements exist between councils of some countries to facilitate the movement of individual doctors, whereas between others additional examinations or evidence has to be provided. Most countries have provision for employing doctors who are non-specialists

Academic training

Many countries offer specific programmes for doctors who wish to combine their medical training with research, education or leadership/management development. The most common programmes focus on clinical or laboratory-based research, typically giving opportunities for doctors in training to step out of clinical training for a period of time or to extend their training whilst studying for a doctorate or master's degree alongside clinical practice.

Internship

While differences exist between countries as to the structure and length of medical education, most require new medical graduates to undertake a period of supervised practice (typically 1 or 2 years) often with a limited scope of registration. This period of internship is typically structured around clinical placements in a small range of core clinical specialties: medicine, surgery and primary care. Because doctors also need skills in assessing and managing patients with acute, undifferentiated presentation, many internship programmes also include an emergency medicine rotation.

Other rotations are highly variable between programmes and jurisdictions, and may include paediatrics, reproductive health, mental health and community placements. Progression from internship normally requires satisfactory completion of formal assessments, often with a strong emphasis on workplace-based assessment, but some include written assessment.

In the US however, the majority of graduates from medical school progress into residency speciality training programmes. This initially reflected that American students were graduate entrants in medical school and therefore already more mature, and traditionally the students had a higher level of patient contact and management exposure prior to graduation.

Speciality training

Specialty training is where doctors become a specific 'type' of doctor, such as surgeon, psychiatrist or 'general practitioner' (GP, family doctor). The length of speciality training ranges from 3 to 10 years depending on the specialty and country/region. In high income countries (e.g. Canada, UK, US) around 60 specialities and subspecialties exist. In LMICs, the number of subspecialties tends to be much lower because health services are less specialised, there are fewer qualified specialists and subsequently a lack of training posts. In order to address this, agreements with other countries have been established to train doctors in required specialties (e.g. surgery, family medicine), who then return to their home country to practise. As in undergraduate education, specialty training may also have a focus on acquiring knowledge and skills that will enable the practitioner to function at an advanced level in rural, remote or relatively under-resourced settings.

Each specialty generally has its own set of national educational standards and assessments, administered by a professional body that is distinct from the overall medical regulator (and may also be distinct from providers of undergraduate education, e.g. professional boards or medical colleges). Specialty training posts are often strictly controlled at national level, tied to workforce planning and the future needs of the healthcare system. Once a doctor has undergone the relevant clinical experience and passed examinations, they become eligible for the specialist register and can gain a post as a consultant or specialist. Hodges and others have critiqued the 'time-served' apprenticeship model of training, suggesting that moving towards competency-based and more tailored personalised training may be more appropriate to address individuals' different rates of learning and experience (Hodges and Lingard, 2012).

Continuing professional development

Once qualified and registered in their field, most countries require doctors to engage in (and be able to evidence) a commitment to education throughout their career in the form of continuing professional development (CPD) or medical education (CME). The main purpose of CPD is for doctors to keep up to date with evolving knowledge and procedures, and to ensure safe practice. Engagement in CPD is typically through participation in small, accredited training/educational courses that are assigned 'points' or 'credits'. The number of credits is broadly correlated with the time taken to complete the activity. Increasingly, evidence of CPD participation is a requirement for relicensing (or revalidation). Relicensing is typically undertaken on a 3 to 5-year cycle. It sometimes involves examinations but generally is carried out using a portfolio of evidence.

3 Evidence-guided education

Table 3.1 Comparison between methodologies

	Qualitative	Quantitative	Mixed methods
Assumptions	Constructivist Interpretive Inductive	Positivist Deductive	Pragmatist
Research questions	Exploratory Broad Seek understanding Describe Provide insights	Specific Narrow Hypothetical Test theories Determine Relate Cause Significance	
Inquiry approaches	Grounded theory Phenomenology Ethnography Case studies Narrative	Surveys Experiments Numerical data analysis	Mix
Data collection	Unstructured/semistructured interviews Focus groups Open-ended questions Texts Observation	Structured interviews Closed questions Numbers Online polls Randomised controlled trials	Mix of both, e.g. either: quantitative first to define interview topic; or qualitative first to define survey questions
Data analysis	Thematic Discourse	Statistical tests	
Considerations	Less generalisable Trustworthiness Reflexivity	Validity Reliability Confounding variables	

Source: adapted from Creswell, 2009.

Box 3.1 Interviews

- **Structured:** questions and areas to explore are set prior to the interview. They are explored in order. Less commonly used in qualitative approaches.
- **Semistructured:** broad questions and areas to explore are set in advance but not necessarily covered in order. The interviewer explores more areas in depth depending on the interviewee's answers and may add extra areas as appropriate to probe more deeply.
- **Unstructured:** used in narrative approaches. The interviewer begins with an invitation to the interviewee to tell their story or describe an experience.

Box 3.2 Effectiveness reviews

Effectiveness reviews aim to gather, analyse and synthesise findings across multiple studies to provide evidence of whether a particular educational method, process or intervention is effective, why it is effective, how it produced outcomes etc. Rarely is there a simple 'yes or no' answer but findings may suggest a trend towards a particular approach in certain contexts. These reviews will probably include quantitative and qualitative data. Occasionally, meta-analysis of quantitative data may be possible. Narrative approaches may be appropriate for qualitative data and mixed methods for realist reviews.

Medical Education at a Glance, First Edition. Edited by Judy McKimm, Kirsty Forrest and Jill Thistlethwaite © 2017 John Wiley & Sons, Ltd. Published 2017 by John Wiley & Sons, Ltd.

The **evidence-based practice** (EBP) (or evidence-based medicine, EBM) approach to healthcare delivery recommends that all clinical decisions and management plans should have evidence to support them. Similarly in medical education, best practice would be that learning, teaching and assessment are developed and implemented based on evidence of effectiveness. However, education is a complex endeavour and evidence is contextual, therefore a more pragmatic process is that of evidence-guided (or evidence-informed) education. Educators sift and appraise available evidence and consider how this may relate to their contexts such as the mix of learners, numbers, resources and defined learning outcomes. They then apply what they have learned from the evidence to their local situation.

Compared with clinical practice, medical education research and evaluation is a fairly recent field. There are fewer systematic reviews and the gold standard of evidence derived from randomised clinical trials (RCTs) is not generally feasible, or appropriate, for education. There is also a diversity of epistemologies (the origin and nature of knowledge) and methodologies that can be bewildering to the novice.

The nature of evidence

The meaning of evidence depends on the purpose we use it for and the context in which it is applied. Evidence may be empirical, theoretical, or experiential: 'A pluralistic approach to evidence calls for choices to be made about the purpose to which evidence is to be put, the type of source material, the key stakeholders who are considered, and the relationship between empirical evidence and theory' (Thistlethwaite *et al.*, 2012a p.454).

Research and evaluation

The question that funders and medical programme leaders frequently ask is: is this education, course or training effective? In other words, what is the value of our interventions? Educators, therefore, are involved extensively in evaluation. The NHS (UK) distinguishes between **research** and **evaluation**, though both generate 'evidence'.

Research: 'the attempt to derive generalisable new knowledge, including studies that aim to generate hypotheses as well as studies that aim to test them'

Evaluation: 'is designed and conducted solely to define or judge current care' – and we may substitute education for care in this definition (Health Research Authority, 2013).

Much evaluation is outcomes focussed: did learners learn? What did they learn? However we also need to know how and why learners learn or don't learn? Patton (2008) writes that evaluation poses the questions: 'What? So what? Now what?' Realist evaluation poses a different set: 'What works, for whom, in what circumstances, in what respects, to what extent and why' (Pawson and Tilley, 1997), stressing the importance of context. What might be effective in a medical school with 100 students per year may not translate so well to one with 500 in a cohort.

Evaluation is important for institutions in the pursuit of quality; good quality evaluation may have a wider audience if it encompasses both outcomes and process and is potentially applicable in other contexts. The methods used for the collection of evidence for evaluation and research are similar. A frequently used model for evaluation in health professional education, the *Kirkpatrick Framework* (Kirkpatrick and Kirkpatrick, 2006), is described in Chapter 10.

Quantitative and qualitative data

Research methodologies are broadly divided into two types: **quantitative** (generating numerical and statistical data) and **qualitative** (generating observations and texts such as interview transcripts for interpretation). Frequently, a combination of the two is appropriate – mixed methods (Table 3.1).

Quantitative approaches

The underlying premise is positivism, with the assumption that reality is fixed and measurable. Research questions focus on how many, how much and how often. The process is primarily hypothesis driven and deductive. Numbers of participants are usually large to generate statistically valid and generalisable results. Methods of data collection include surveys, structured questionnaires, closed questions, rating and attitudinal scales, comparison of groups (horizontal or longitudinal) and randomisation (though this is difficult and has ethical issues in education). In education, quantitative approaches are used, for example to compare participants before and after an intervention, measuring change in knowledge, skills and performance.

Qualitative approaches

Frequently perceived erroneously by novices from a biomedical tradition as being less rigorous than quantitative research, qualitative research is based on the assumption that reality is socially constructed and negotiated. Research questions focus on explanation, why and how. The process is primarily theory generating and inductive. Participant numbers are frequently small. Methods of data collection include semistructured and unstructured interviews, focus groups, open and free text questionnaires, observation (ethnography), case studies and narratives. Analysis includes textual (hermeneutics), thematic and discourse. Grounded theory is a specific methodology that now includes different approaches. As a number of ways of carrying out data analysis are available, researchers should explain the rationale behind their chosen approach in order to ensure the trustworthiness of their findings. In education, qualitative approaches are used to explore participants' feelings, experience and understanding, as well as the phenomena of the education process.

Realist approaches

Realism is situated between the quantitative and qualitative paradigms, between positivism and social constructionism (Thistlethwaite, 2015a). It focuses on causation in complex systems, through an exploration of mechanisms acting in contexts to produce outcomes: the C-M-O relationship (Pawson and Tilley, 1997). Realist evaluation requires a mixed methodology (see also Chapter 10).

Systematic reviews

The medical and health professional education journals are a good source of reviews of education (e.g. Barr *et al.*, 1999, 2000), as is the Best Evidence Medical and Health Professional Education (BEME) collaboration: www.bemecollaboration.org. (Now known as Best Evidence Health Professional Education.) These reviews comprehensively critically appraise the evidence supplied by primary sources in the published literature on a particular topic. They identify gaps, flaws and further research questions, while synthesising the evidence for trends to guide and inform education.

4 Learning theories: paradigms and orientations

Practice points

- Learning theories draw from a range of subject disciplines
- Perspectives on learning influence our practice as educators, both tacitly and overtly
- Orientations to learning tend to focus primarily on the individual or on social processes
- Understanding such orientations and their underpinning paradigms is essential to provide relevant learning experiences

Figure 4.1 Orientations on learning. Source: adapted from Mann *et al*., 2011.

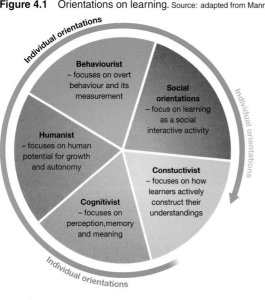

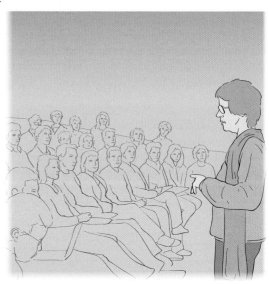

Table 4.1 Three paradigms underpinning learning and research activities

Positivist	Postpositivist/Pragmatist	Constructivist/Interpretivist
Seeks universal, generalisable 'truths'	Critical realist: critical of ability to be certain of reality	No universal rules exist
Knowledge is derived from observed phenomena	Knowledge is derived from triangulating across multiple, competing perspectives	Knowledge is created through an active learning process, interconnectedness and social negotiation
Knowledge is absolute, external to learner and measurable	Knowledge is constructed: it evolves through variation, selection and retention	Knowledge is constructed based on personal experiences, culture, and context
Objectivity essential and possible by individuals	Position/bias of researcher/teacher needs to be acknowledged	Individuals actively create their subjective representations of objective reality
Knowledge can be transmitted as it 'is'	Some theories/ideas stand the test of time through 'natural selection'	Knowledge is constructed from learner's previous knowledge, not acquired; language and learning are inextricably intertwined
Scientific method collects evidence through observation, measurement, experimentation, empirical	Scientific reasoning and common-sense reasoning are similar; mixed methods of research Important to recognise theory-laden observations and methods, and limitation of scientific method	Collects and interprets data through primarily qualitative methods, collaborative research with participants, identifies position of researcher/ teacher, brings values into the research
Wants to discover 'how things really work' and 'how things really are' in order to predict and control	Goal of science is to try to define reality, whilst acknowledging all measurements are fallible and contain error	Aims to explain and interpret different realities from the perspective of those being studied in order to deepen understanding
Emotions, morals, values and beliefs can't be studied as not measurable	If recognise own world-view and theoretical stance, then can study emotions, values, beliefs etc.	Values, beliefs, meaning are central to understanding how people function and can all be studied
Key theorists: Skinner, Pavlov, Comte, Durkheim	Key theorists: Popper, Kuhm, Habermas, Gagne, Ausubel	Key theorists: Vygotsky, Dewey, Bruner, Piaget,

Source: adapted from Trochim, 2006.

Medical Education at a Glance, First Edition. Edited by Judy McKimm, Kirsty Forrest and Jill Thistlethwaite © 2017 John Wiley & Sons, Ltd. Published 2017 by John Wiley & Sons, Ltd.

This chapter summarises some of the educational philosophies and paradigms underpinning how we envisage learning taking place. An understanding of these provides guidance as to which activities might best facilitate effective learning in various contexts, helps us understand why people struggle, and facilitates the selection of relevant curricula and course design, teaching, learning and assessment methods, and research and evaluation strategies. We provide a summary of some of the most dominant orientations to learning used in medical education (Figure 4.1) and provide suggestions for further reading on this extensive, shifting and often polarising topic.

Philosophies and paradigms

Before we look at the perspectives or theories themselves, it is important to consider the philosophical underpinnings of the nature of reality and knowledge. An educator or researcher's philosophical position will determine how they see reality and how they perceive knowledge. Ontology considers the nature and form of reality. Epistemology considers the 'study or a theory of the nature and grounds of knowledge especially with reference to its limits and validity' (Merriam online dictionary, 2016). Methodology focuses on the specific ways that we can use to understand our world better.

The three paradigms in Table 4.1 show a continuum from a positivist approach through to a more interpretivist approach. Scientific paradigms comprise sets of theories, concepts and thought patterns. In social sciences, a paradigm is more like a way of thinking about or perspective on the world – a worldview. Over time, and in disciplines, dominant paradigms exist (such as outcomes-based education) and sometimes paradigm shifts occur, where a new way of conceptualising the world is taken, for example competency-based education.

If a *real* world is assumed, then a positivist approach will be taken, knowledge will be seen as *true*, measurable and transmittable. In contrast, a constructivist or interpretivist standpoint would see *reality* as subjective, constantly being mediated and constructed through interactions of agents (Lincoln *et al.*, 2011). Knowledge is therefore seen as co-constructed and created, based on an individual's prior experiences, culture and the learning environment (Table 4.1).

This is important for educators (and learners) because the way we see the world will affect and influence the way we think learning happens, and subsequently the methods we use to teach and facilitate (and research) learning. In education, being able to look through different 'lenses' or take different perspectives is helpful, because then we can select relevant learning, teaching and assessment methods for our learners. For example, a more positivist lens can be useful when teaching or assessing a body of agreed knowledge, such as human anatomy. We can teach and assess these 'facts' (whilst acknowledging that that there are still things we don't know yet) as there is agreement that, say, a femur is a femur. If we are teaching other topics, for example health beliefs, then taking a constructivist or interpretivist approach will be helpful because beliefs are culturally and individually derived. We want our learners to understand this so that they can adapt their practice to the needs and beliefs of individual patients.

Orientations to learning

Merriam *et al.* (2007) set out five orientations to learning (Figure 4.1), which can be grouped into those that focus on the individual and those that focus on social processes. We have mentioned constructivism already, which is a broad philosophical position or paradigm as well as a learning orientation in which learners need to be supported in making meaning through integrating knowledge, beliefs and experiences.

Behaviourist

This orientation focuses on observable, measurable behaviours, typically seen as responses to external stimuli, rather than what is going on in the mind. Learning occurs in the way the response is rewarded or sanctioned (through conditioning and reinforcement of acceptable behaviours) as explained by psychologists including Watson, Skinner, Pavlov and Thorndike, who initially worked with animals. In education, a behaviourist orientation is reflected in the use of behavioural objectives, provision of feedback to improve performance and the development of practical skills through deliberate practice with expert feedback.

Cognitive

Covert processes, or acts of mind, such as processing perceptions, making meaning of events, memory, problem-solving, creativity, attention and language use are the focus. Drawing initially from the idea of the brain as a computer, memory is seen as an active processor of information and knowledge. Cognitive neuroscience and experimental psychologists, such as Piaget, Miller and Bruner, contributed to the way in which behaviours are mediated by the mind. In education, applications include meta-cognition, transfer of learning and instructional design.

Social

Social Learning Theory suggests that, through observation and feedback, the learner extracts information from the environment about performance expectations (Bandura, 1977). Social Cognitive Theory brings the social, behaviourist and cognitive approaches together so that 'our actions, learning and functioning are the result of a continuous, dynamic, reciprocal interaction between three sets of determinants: personal, environmental (situational) and behavioural' (Kauffman and Mann, 2014, p. 9). These theories assume that humans have five basic capabilities: symbolising, forethought, vicarious, self-regulatory and self-reflective, and have the capacity for self-efficacy (Bandura, 1977). Kauffman and Mann suggest that a social cognitive theory approach leads us to incorporate these learning processes into curricula and teaching:

- Formulation of clear objectives, goals or outcomes
- Modelling or demonstration of tasks and behaviours
- Provision of task-relevant knowledge
- Guided practice and feedback
- Opportunities for reflection.

Transformative learning theories (e.g. Mezirow, 1991) also consider learning as a social process. Through critical thinking, exposure to alternative viewpoints, reflection and discourse, learners are empowered to develop new paradigms, assumptions and ways of being.

Humanist

The humanist perspective draws heavily from social psychologists such as Maslow and Rogers who emphasise the importance of enabling learners to learn for themselves and become intrinsically motivated to achieve autonomy and self-actualisation (reaching full potential). Self-directed and experiential learning activities, which aim to develop independence, are seen as fundamental for personal growth.

5 Learning theories and clinical practice

Practice points

- Facilitating learning in the clinical setting is complex and challenging
- Sociocultural and work-based learning theorists provide explanatory frameworks, which can help teachers design relevant learning activities
- Meaningful learning experiences are provided through participating in work activities, but this can be problematic

Table 5.1 Central concepts of Engeström's Third Generation Activity Theory (Engeström, 2007)

Concepts	Concept explanation
1 Co-configuration	Changing and reciprocal relationships among actors in the system result in *a joined-up* performance of a task or provision of service, which may result in more effective ways of working or learning
2 Knotworking	Considers the fluid and changing membership of groups and the constant improvisation that may be required in learning groups and service delivery, e.g. learning *at the bedside,* in multidisciplinary teams
3 Expansive learning	New ways of working and thinking created or constructed *on the fly* exposing all professionals to change, expanding understandings and enriching practices
4 Boundary crossing	A focus on actual or reported practices, which illustrate the professionals' negotiation and renegotiation of ways of working and the extent to which they may work within the discursive practices of others, e.g. physicians' associates or advanced practice nurses working to the medical model

Source: adapted from Barrow *et al.,* 2015.

Figure 5.1 Scaffolding and the ZPD

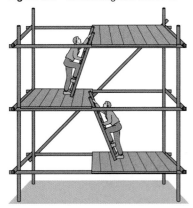

Vygotsky, a Russian educational psychologist, talked about learning that could be achieved by the input of a teacher (but which the learner could not achieve on their own) as taking place in the Zone of Proximal Development (ZPD) (Vygotsky 1978). For learners to learn effectively in the ZPD requires teachers to put activities in place to help the learner to apply what they already know to the current topic being discussed. This is known as 'educational scaffolding' and without it the learner does not have links or links that are sufficiently strong within their cognitive structure to be able to apply relevant knowledge (even though it exists somewhere in their memory). Scaffolding can be verbal (through feedback, giving hints, questioning, instructing and explaining); procedural (use of teaching and learning techniques such as small group work, case-based learning) or instructional (programme design, access to learning materials).

Table 5.2 Perspectives on learning

Perspectives on learning	Key principles

Adult learning (*andragogy*)	Adults are seen as learning differently from children because they have:
	    a need to know
	    motivation to learn
	    a readiness to learn.
	The learners' self-concept is important; it can enhance or impede learning
	Learners' previous experiences of learning, background and culture affect learning
	Individuals have different orientations to learning, which need to be taken account of
	Critics of adult learning suggest that adults and children learn in similar ways and the distinction is unhelpful

Self-directed learning or directed self-learning	Where the teacher provides help and direction to learners (scaffolding) but the learner takes responsibility for their individual learning Depending on the situation and learner's needs, teacher control and individual autonomy will vary Professionals need to be self-directed and take responsibility for their own learning
Lifelong learning	Learning continues throughout life Assumes a complex, ever-changing body of knowledge and technologies Learners need to be equipped with the tools and techniques needed to learn through their career Learners therefore need *transferable* skills: to appraise knowledge, think critically, be adaptive and open to change so they can navigate an uncertain world and future
Adaptive or differentiated learning	The learning cohort is not an homogenous group Learners learn at different rates and in different ways Curricula and learning tailored to individual needs will enable learners to achieve standards or competences at different rates Digital technologies provide opportunities for adaptive, individually tailored learning

In this chapter we consider some theories, perspectives and practices that are particularly influential in medical education in the clinical (work-based) context. Whilst facilitating learning in the classroom setting has its own challenges, the workplace is much more complex, particularly as its primary purpose is to deliver a service and care for patients, not to ensure learning occurs.

Sociocultural theory

Like social–cognitive theory, this theory also considers the individual learner within the diversity of their social context, but here learning is much more culturally located, influenced and mediated by culturally constructed artefacts (such as language, dress codes, rituals and technologies), which mediate learning. Vygotsky (1978) considered what the role and activities of the teacher should be in facilitating learning (Figure 5.1). Other writers focus on wider aspects of culture such as communities or systems.

Communities of practice

Conceptualised by Lave and Wenger (1991) and developed further by other theorists, communities of practice (CoP) situates learning integrally within the social practices of a community. The community has specific ways of learning and practices that facilitate the development of a learner on a trajectory from novice to expert practitioner through a process of legitimate peripheral participation (LPP). The status of being a *learner* enables individuals to participate in activities that they would not be allowed to do otherwise, for example being able to observe a consultation, undertake an intimate examination or assist in an operation. Participation in these social relationships and processes help learners develop technical skills and knowledge (*formal* learning). They also strongly influence the more informal or implicit processes involved in identity formation: *becoming* and *being* a doctor.

Activity theory

Developed from Vygotsky and colleagues' work, activity theory locates learning by individual agents within social, collective systems. 'It is also concerned with social or cultural transformation, drawing on the complexities, multiple perspectives and conflicts within social practices to promote cultural change' (Barrow *et al.,* 2015). The components of an activity system interact dynamically, individual and collective learning occurs through the way in which activities mediate between individuals and their social worlds (Tsui *et al.,* 2009); see Table 5.1 for some central concepts from Engeström's (2007) work in relation to learning in the clinical context, where service and education intersect.

Work-based learning

Some writers believe that applying formal educational models to the complex, dynamic world of work is unhelpful (Billett, 2004; Swanwick, 2005). Work-based learning theorists therefore draw more heavily on social learning and sociocultural theories to explain what is occurring and identify practice implications. Perspectives such as industrial relations and sociological theories offer additional insights into how learning happens at work (Morris and Blaney, 2014). Learning activities also have to be designed in terms of the relationship between learning and work, for example is it learning *for* work, learning *at* work or learning *from* work (Seagraves and Boyd, 1996).

Billett (2004) suggests that work-based learning is essentially participatory, and it is through active participation that learning happens. Engagement of learners in relevant participatory practices is therefore essential. However, because the workplace is primarily about work practices and activities (rather than learning), participatory practices can be contested between *newcomers* who want to learn and *old timers* who fear displacement and regulate learning (Lave and Wenger, 1991). Billett notes that the workplace must therefore be invitational through identifying affordances to learners to participate in (and therefore learn from) work-based practices.

Perspectives on learning

Mann *et al.* (2011) suggest that dominant perspectives on professional development and practice include adult learning, self-directed learning and lifelong learning, we would add adaptive or differentiated learning. Table 5.2 sets out their key features. Whilst each has a different focus, they all draw from assumptions that learners are individuals who learn in context through experience and reflection, and need to be motivated to learn (intrinsically or extrinsically).

Experiential learning

The idea that learning occurs through experience is central to medical education. It is reflected in curriculum design that provides meaningful clinical learning opportunities and teaching and learning practices that are aligned with learning outcomes or competences, are learner centred and relevant to the stage of education and training. Experiential learning theory suggests that learning is best achieved when individuals *actively engage* with authentic experiences in a content domain, and then *reflect* on those experiences to derive relevance (abstraction) they can test in other contexts. Kolb's experiential learning cycle (1984) expands on the constructivist foundations established by Dewey (1933), who theorised that the successive processes of interaction, reflection and abstraction of concepts led to better understanding and retention over time. Kolb also suggested that analytical skills were necessary for conceptualisation and that a process of active experimentation to test those abstractions was essential for acquiring expertise.

Simulation based education

In clinical practice, opportunities for reflection and experimentation are limited, and concerns about patient safety are paramount. Simulation-based education (SBE) is one way of providing an experiential environment in which learners and clinicians can acquire, refine, and maintain their abilities in contextually relevant situations, without impacting patient or clinician safety. Best practices in SBE utilise deliberate practice coupled with a deliberate process for reflection (Ericsson *et al.,* 1993). This furthers connections between theory and practice, the transfer of learning to other areas of professional experience and development for individuals and teams (see Chapters 19, 20 and 26).

6 The curriculum

Practice points

- A curriculum defines the intended programme of learning, underpinned by a clear educational philosophy
- All elements need to be aligned to facilitate effective learning
- Factors influencing curriculum development and delivery vary over time, according to individual learners' and society's needs

Table 6.1 Trends in medical education curriculum planning and design: Flexner, SPICES and PRISMS

Flexner (1910)	Harden *et al.* (1984): the SPICES model	Bligh *et al.* (2001): PRISMS
Teacher centred	Student centred	Practice based linked with professional development
Knowledge giving	Problem based	Relevant to students and communities
Discipline led	Integrated	Interprofessional and interdisciplinary
Hospital oriented	Community oriented	Shorter courses taught in smaller units
Standard programme	Electives (+ core)	Multisite locations
Opportunistic (apprenticeship)	Systematic	Symbiotic (organic whole)

Figure 6.1 Curriculum alignment. Source: adapted from Biggs, 1999.

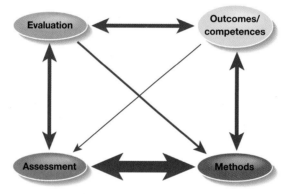

Figure 6.2 Not just one curriculum.

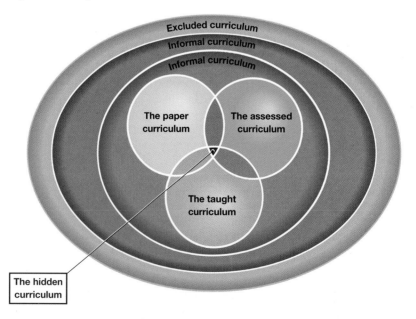

Medical Education at a Glance, First Edition. Edited by Judy McKimm, Kirsty Forrest and Jill Thistlethwaite © 2017 John Wiley & Sons, Ltd. Published 2017 by John Wiley & Sons, Ltd.

Acurriculum is a statement of the intended aims and objectives, content, experiences, outcomes and processes of an educational programme including:

• A description of the training structure (entry requirements, length and organisation of the programme, including its flexibilities, and assessment system)

• A description of expected methods of learning, teaching, feedback and supervision.

The curriculum should cover both generic professional and specialty specific areas. The word curriculum derives from the Latin *currere* meaning 'to run'. This implies that one of the functions of a curriculum is to provide a template or design that enables learning to take place. Curricula usually define the learning that is expected to take place during a course or programme of study in terms of knowledge, skills and attitudes/behaviours. They should specify the main teaching, learning and assessment methods as well as provide an indication of the learning resources required to support the effective delivery of the course. By contrast, the syllabus describes the content of a programme and is one part of a curriculum. Most curricula are not developed *de novo* and all operate within organisational and societal constraints.

Curriculum in context

The educational and professional context must be discussed and clearly defined before a curriculum can be designed and delivered. This can reflect a number of factors: current or prevailing educational or social ideology; organisational culture; politics; economy; students', teachers', communities' and service users' views; employers and other stakeholders; professional and regulatory bodies; funding bodies and history or influence of the past. In any discipline, trends in general education and specific trends or issues in medical or healthcare education that relate to the healthcare system or context will need to be addressed. Power relations between different 'tribes and territories' (Becher and Trowler, 2001) need to be acknowledged and worked with or around. The organisational infrastructure will also affect curriculum options, for example the IT infrastructure, proximity of clinical locations to where students live and study, type and number of clinical placements, physical facilities and human resources.

Educational philosophy and theories

Aside from practical issues, depending on the stance and backgrounds of those involved, the educational philosophy, curriculum design and priorities of the programme will be influenced by different perspectives on learning. These may include adult learning, student-centred learning, active learning, self-directed learning, workplace learning and competency-based approaches (see Chapters 4 and 5). These approaches are themselves underpinned by educational theories or paradigms including behaviourism; cognitivism; constructivist, social learning and situational theories; humanist and motivational theories; identity theories, and descriptive and other theories (e.g. affordances, activity theory, communities of practice) (see Chapter 5). An ideal curriculum will not be dominated by any one perspective or approach but will select appropriate learning activities to best facilitate learning in different contexts by a range of learners with varying needs and preferences.

Curriculum alignment

Biggs (1999) introduced the idea of curriculum alignment in that all aspects of the curriculum need to form an integrated whole. In other words, the specified outcomes, objectives or competencies need to be aligned with relevant learning and teaching approaches; and assessed by relevant assessment methods (see Chapters 38–43) with the evaluation strategy utilising data from a range of sources (see Chapters 3 and 10). The benefits of curriculum alignment are that clarity of the curriculum is promoted, everything is transparent to both learners and teachers and, because all of the components are inextricably linked, deep learning is encouraged. Outcomes-based education utilises an aligned approach to curriculum design and delivery as does the 'spiral curriculum', in which topics are purposefully repeated in increasing depth to reinforce learning.

Curriculum structure and approach

In basic (undergraduate) medical education, the overall design or structure of the curriculum has changed over time from one which was totally apprenticeship based to one which is partly university and partly clinically based, although the proportion varies between curricula (see Chapter 2). The traditional curriculum (primarily designed for school leavers) comprises 2 or 3 early years spent studying preclinical subjects (primarily sciences) at university followed by 2 to 4 years in the clinical setting. In the US and Canada, but also in other countries in Europe and Australia, graduate-entry medicine is undertaken following a premedical or earlier relevant degree programme. This curriculum is usually 4 years in duration.

Practice-ready graduates

Since the early 1990s, in a drive to ensure graduates are more practice ready, a number of changes have occurred. Curricula have become more integrated so that, rather than studying subject disciplines (e.g. physiology) or clinical specialities in isolation, the programme is structured around body systems (e.g. cardiovascular), patient problems or cases. Clinical experience with patient contact is introduced earlier and biomedical sciences are revisited later in the course so as to help contextualise learning. In many countries, exposure to community based or community-engaged learning, particularly in rural and remote areas, is included in the programme to both enhance clinical experience and encourage recruitment to underserved areas. Most programmes also provide opportunities for electives (i.e. student choices), which may be in other countries with different health systems, in areas of medicine students might wish to specialise in, or areas of interest, including research, overseas electives and community projects.

Approaches such as problem-based, case-based learning and team-based learning (PBL, CBL and TBL), are used in some medical programmes as it is felt they help facilitate learning whilst preparing graduates for clinical practice (see Chapter 31). Competency-based curricula are increasingly widespread, particularly in postgraduate education and training. Reflecting wider educational change and the flexibility of mobile technologies, the flipped classroom or inverted curriculum, places emphasis on assimilating background knowledge before the students meet other students or/and a teacher. The face-to-face time is then used for questioning, critical analysis, developing understanding, discussion and reflection. This approach provides opportunities for more self-directed learning of 'facts' by students, with the classroom being used much more purposefully (Hurtubise *et al.*, 2015).

7 Planning and design

Figure 7.1 Example lesson plan

Workshop: Opportunistic clinical teaching
Aims: To improve understanding of what makes good opportunistic clinical teaching

Timing (min)	Teacher activity	Student Activity	Resources
5	Introduction	Listening	
10	What you are hoping to get from the workshop?	Participating	
15	Background to clinical teaching	Listening	PowerPoint
15	What challenges/ problems have you faced concerning clinical teaching?	Buzz groups	
15	Feed back to large group	Participating	Flip charts
10	What the literature says	Listening	PowerPoint
10	Break	Break	
15	What have you seen that Addresses these challenges/ problems?	Buzz groups	
15	Feed back to large group	Participating	Flip charts
10	What the literature says	Listening	PowerPoint
5	Summary/close	Take away literature pack Evaluation forms	

Figure 7.3 Designing a course

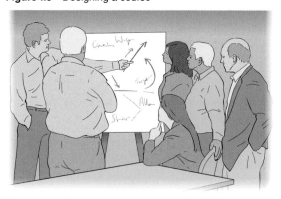

Figure 7.4 The educational cycle

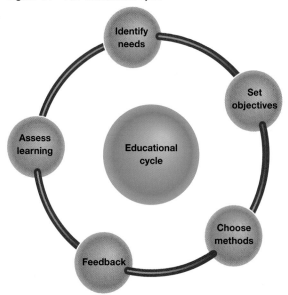

Figure 7.2 Sample timetable

Time/Day	Monday	Tuesday	Wednesday	Thursday	Friday
9.00–10.00		Lecture – Psychology of ageing			Lecture – Asking permission and keeping confidentiality
10.00–11.00	Problem Based Learning Tutorial	Lecture – Theories of ageing	Self-directed learning	Problem Based Learning Tutorial	Lecture – Introduction to nutrition and nutritional deficiency
11.00–12.00		Lecture – Looking after older people in the community			Lecture – Depression and bereavement
Lunch					
13.00–15.00		Clinical Skills – Principles of manual handling			
15.00–17.00	Visit to local residential home	Communication Skills – Communication with older people	GP Visits – Older person home visits	Self-directed learning	Self-directed learning

Source: Figure 7.1, 7.2 *Essential Guide to Generic Skills*. Copyright © 2006 Nicola Cooper, Kirsty Forrest and Paul Cramp. Published by Blackwell Publishing Ltd. Reproduced with permission of Kirsty Forrest.

Medical Education at a Glance, First Edition. Edited by Judy McKimm, Kirsty Forrest and Jill Thistlethwaite © 2017 John Wiley & Sons, Ltd. Published 2017 by John Wiley & Sons, Ltd.

Whether you are developing a single learning event or a whole degree programme, taking time to design and plan carefully is essential. Curriculum or programme design reflects the principles discussed in Chapter 6, which enable you to decide on your overall approach and underpinning pedagogy (teaching/learning methods or practice) and give a structure and coherence to the programme. More detailed planning is then important because it allows you to test out whether the approach and ideas will work in practice. For example, if you want to incorporate small group case or problem-based learning sessions, then you will need appropriately equipped learning spaces and trained facilitators. If these are unavailable or only available at certain times of the day/week then you may have to redesign your programme to fit within these constraints or change your learning approach (Figure 7.1 and 7.2).

Components of course or lesson planning

The principles of design and planning are the same whether at programme level or for an individual teaching event, in that the key elements need to be identified, agreed and written down (Table 7.1). Learners and staff involved in teaching and administration all need to be very clear about the language used when explaining the principles and different elements of the programme to avoid confusion.

There is less reliance on defining highly specific behavioural objectives now, and an emerging focus (particularly in postgraduate education) on a competency-based curriculum, which specifies the professional attributes and skills that graduates and doctors should display. Whilst technically the terms are different, in practice, the terms objectives, outcomes and competences are often used interchangeably. More recent thinking (e.g. by Caverzagie *et al.*, 2015) define what should be learned in clinical practice as entrustable professional activities (EPAs). These activities are defined professional practice tasks or responsibilities that will be entrusted to a learner once sufficient specific competence is reached to allow for unsupervised practice. However, despite the jargon, 'what is important is fitness for purpose, and the main purposes of stating the intended learning achievements of the curriculum are:

- To inform learners of what they should achieve
- To inform teachers about what they should help learners to achieve
- To be the basis of the assessment system, so that everyone knows what will be assessed

- To reflect accurately the nature of the profession into which the learner is being inducted and the professional characteristics that must be acquired' (Grant, 2014, p. 41).

It is not just in face-to-face learning where all course components need to be aligned; learning materials, library and online support all have to be constructed to help the learner achieve the specified outcomes of the training programme. In addition there should be relevant and timely simulated and clinical experiences available.

Learners' needs

Whilst learners may be on the same education or training programme, because of their backgrounds, qualifications, experience, interests, personalities and learning preferences, they will have different needs from teachers and from the programme itself. One of the responsibilities of the teacher is to help align the stated, formal learning outcomes with the individual learner's educational needs (Figure 7.4). Assessing learning needs can be done relatively informally at the start of a teaching session simply by asking the learners what they would like to learn or what they expect to get out of the teaching session. Making this a routine part of teaching will help you to meet learners' needs more effectively. Of course, learners do not necessarily know what they need to learn; they may have blind spots.

Hussey and Smith (2003) note that teaching sessions should build in an open space for emergent learning outcomes – outcomes identified by learners which you might not have included in your lesson plan. Spencer (2010) describes other activities concerned with helping clinical teachers to optimise teaching and learning opportunities that arise in daily practice, such as using appropriate questioning techniques and teaching in different clinical contexts. Such techniques often involve discussing learners' performance or understanding with them, and are built into everyday practice.

From the perspective of the programme, it is also important to define what those entering each stage of a programme will need to know and be able to do. For example, potential undergraduates might need to have had healthcare work experience or need to demonstrate understanding of biomedical sciences at a certain level. Newly graduated doctors should be able to perform certain clinical or practical procedures. These will vary depending on the content of the programmes involved and expectations of stakeholders, including employers.

Table 7.1 Definitions of course components

Components	Definition and examples
Aims	Defines what the programme or teacher is trying to achieve overall. It tells participants what the programme or session is about. 'The aim of this session is to practise eliciting a history in pairs and give feedback to one another about what is good and what needs to be improved'
Learning (or instructional) objectives	Learning objectives state the observable and measurable behaviours that learners should exhibit as a result of participating in a learning programme. 'On completion of this session, the learner should be able to obtain a full medical history from an adult with chest pain in less than 15 minutes and record this accurately in the patient's notes'
Learning outcomes	Learning outcomes state broadly what learners should know, be able to do and how they should behave as a result of participation. 'On completion of this session the learner will be able to demonstrate understanding of the key components of a full medical history and be able to take a history from a simulated patient, showing appropriate clinical and communication skills'
Competences	Competences state what the learner should be able to do as a result of a learning programme, in terms of the skills, knowledge and behaviours that comprise professional performance. 'Routinely undertakes structured interviews ensuring that the patient's concerns, expectations and understanding are identified and addressed'
Learning and teaching methods	The ways in which teachers enable learning to occur so that the intended outcomes are achieved. Methods include face to face (e.g. lecturing, small group work), online learning and self-directed learning, see Chapters 13–29.
Assessment	The way in which student performance is measured in terms of knowledge/ understanding; practical and clinical skills and professional behaviours (see Chapters 38–43).
Evaluation	Evaluation is used to measure how well the programme, module, course or session has met its aims and objectives (see Chapter 10). NB in some countries, evaluation means assessment of student performance, i.e. what we have termed 'assessment'.

8 Equality, diversity and inclusivity

Figure 8.1 Intersecting identities

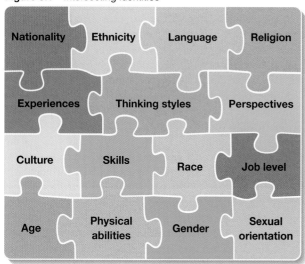

Box 8.1 Inclusive teaching practice

Inclusive teaching practice involves:

- good planning and clear course documentation in different formats;
- a learning environment conducive to learning in terms of layout or accessibility;
- a variety of approaches and methods of learning and assessment;
- setting clear ground rules to encourage participation and respect;
- encouraging engagement through individual, pair and small group work;
- use of culturally appropriate language and examples;
- being willing to challenge prejudice and stereotyping;
- building on learners' diversity as a resource;
- discussion about provision of additional resources as needed.

Figure 8.2 Equality or fairness?

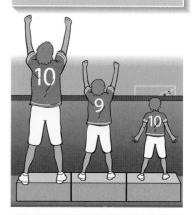

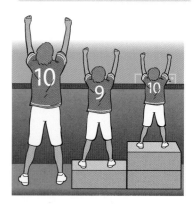

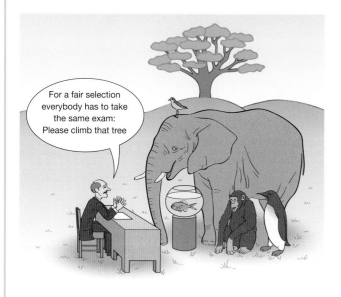

Medical Education at a Glance, First Edition. Edited by Judy McKimm, Kirsty Forrest and Jill Thistlethwaite © 2017 John Wiley & Sons, Ltd. Published 2017 by John Wiley & Sons, Ltd.

We live in a multicultural world in which colleagues, patients, families and communities represent cultural diversity in all its forms. A key responsibility of educators is to ensure learners get the most from their education and training and can achieve their full potential. This requires an understanding of individual learners' needs, how issues or challenges may present in the classroom, and the strategies and options available. As teachers, if we are not careful, addressing equality can simply become a box ticking exercise or we can assume that because university centres or occupational health units exist for working with learners with specific learning needs (e.g. dyspraxia, dyslexia, sensory impairments) or health problems, that their problems will be solved. Utilising pedagogical and organisational approaches that embed equality and diversity into curricular and classroom practices will foster inclusivity at all levels and improve the educational experience of all learners.

Definitions

Equality

The notion of equality is embedded in many countries' legal systems with the overarching aim to try to ensure equality of treatment and fair and open access to opportunities. It is important not to discriminate against someone on the grounds of personal characteristics (such as age, disability, sex, race, religion or belief), which do not impact on eligibility for most occupations or educational experiences. Discrimination, bullying or harassment is also often illegal. In education, selection and assessment processes are increasingly objective and criterion based to help address potential direct or indirect discrimination. Examples include educational interventions or assessments that might directly or indirectly discriminate against groups or individuals from different genders or cultural backgrounds (e.g. Carnes *et al.,* 2015)

Whilst educational institutions have a duty to take reasonable steps to remove disadvantage caused by a characteristic (e.g. adjusting assessment length for a learner with dyslexia; running flexible courses for those with domestic or work commitments), in medicine and other health professions, fitness to practice requirements (e.g. around health, disability or age) defined by regulatory bodies usually outweigh equality legislation. In practical, day-to-day terms, equality means treating everyone fairly and with respect and working with them to help overcome any disadvantage – a form of social justice.

Diversity

Equality legislation provides an underpinning framework and sets out requirements for provision of services but in teaching, we need to do more than this. In practice, classroom diversity is about seeing all learners as individual and different, valuing people's differences and treating them in a way they wish to be treated. This involves holding conversations and building relationships, taking time to hear different stories, valuing different perspectives and using examples and materials representing different cultures or social groups. An approach that welcomes and encourages cultural and social diversity can provide a rich educational experience for all those involved.

However, working with diverse learner groups is not always easy and requires a flexible, culturally relevant approach and practices. Providing safe places for discussion and debate (both in the classroom and outside via social networking or discussion threads) can help teachers introduce and enable constructive discussion of sensitive issues (such as death/dying, race, religion or sexuality) where learners might have very divergent and strong views.

Inclusivity

Recently, there has been a shift from focussing on specific characteristics (such as gender or race) to a more inclusive, intersectional approach that respond to the overlapping, intersecting identities of people, for example as parents, workers, members of religious or other social groups (Higher Education Academy, 2015). This shift helps us move away from what might be seen as a *deficit* approach in which learners require assistance from outside the department (e.g. in specialist units for learners with a disability or for international students), to one in which system, curricular and pedagogical approaches are designed to incorporate *difference*.

An inclusive educational approach aims to give learners a sense of belonging, so that they feel valued and respected for who they are. At the level of the organisation or course planning, this involves taking positive actions to include people from all groups when planning and making decisions.

Challenges

A range of challenges exist in embedding equality and diversity into educational systems, organisations and practices. At system level, much Western research has highlighted the relative lack of female and BME (black and ethnic minority) academics at senior level (e.g. Carr *et al.,* 2015). This gives rise to a lack of role models from diverse backgrounds, exacerbated by a medical student body that, despite widening access interventions, is still predominantly drawn from the higher social classes or higher status social groups (Nicholson and Cleland, 2015). One consequence of this is that cultural practices (such as the length of the working day, timing of meetings and flexibility of course provision) reflect the norms of prevailing social groups. So, considering how systems and organisational practices contribute to creating an inclusive culture is vital.

Privilege

Privilege is a 'special right, advantage or immunity for a particular person' (Pearsall, 2002) or social group. It is culturally derived and can lead to positive discrimination, benefits and favouritism. Understanding that privilege exists can help educators to empower learners differently to achieve their potential and avoid giving privileges that create outliers. For example, rewarding keen and eager students by giving them more time and attention than quieter learners can lead to the quieter learners feeling excluded or marginalised; expecting learners to purchase expensive equipment or books can disadvantage those from poorer backgrounds.

Unconscious bias

'Unconscious bias refers to a bias that we are unaware of, and which happens outside our control. It is a bias that happens automatically and is triggered by our brain making quick judgements and assessments of people and situations, influenced by our background, cultural environment and personal experiences' (ECU, 2013). As educators, we need to accept we all have biases, decide what we will do about this, break the links in our processing (reduce levels of bias) and ensure policies and processes are designed to mitigate the impact of bias wherever possible (ECU, 2013). This is done by challenging stereotypes, being aware of in-groups and out-groups and changing perceptions of out-group members and becoming an 'active bystander' (i.e. notice what is going on around you and intervening or providing help where needed). 'Active bystanders' are important in 'preventing, refocusing, interpreting, mitigating, stopping, remediating and reporting unacceptable behaviour' (Scully and Rowe, 2009).

Principles of selection

Practice points

- The selection process aims to identify people suitable for practice as a doctor and exclude those who are deemed unsuitable
- Selection is typically based on a combination of academic attainment and performance at interview or in a written assessment
- Some schools do not interview; the process is based on academic attainment and a random allocation
- More objective tests are being introduced into selection such as the Multiple Mini Interview (MMI) and the Situational Judgement Test (SJT)

Figure 9.1 Examples of selection processes

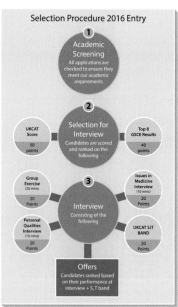

Figure 9.2 Anytown Mini Multiple Interview

Station 1

You are just about to go into a lecture where attendance is monitored when one of your friends asks you to sign in for them as they have to go to return an overdue library book.

What do you say?

Station 2

You are on placement with a final year student who you'd heard on the grapevine has anorexia. You hear her vomiting in the toilets and when you ask her if she is OK, she says she is fine.

Who do you speak to?

Station 3

Your second year case study project was with Annie, a terminally ill cancer patient. In the course of the project, you got very close to her and a few months later, you are informed that she has left you some money in their will 'in recognition of your care and compassion'.

What issues does this identify?

Is there a difference between being a student or a qualified doctor?

Station 4

At this station you are asked to have a conversation with this patient (actor) for four minutes and find out six things about them. A bell will ring and then you will be asked to recall these and answer questions about them.

Station 5

Tell us about a time when you found yourself in a dilemma. What was the dilemma, what issues did this raise for you and what did you do?

What learning lessons did the experience give you?

Station 6

You are on placement with Dr Jan, a GP who tells you that he often gives antibiotics or other unnecessary medication to some patients 'because it makes them feel better and they expect him to give them medicine'.

What do you think about Dr Jan's practice?

What would you do, if anything?

Station 7

What attracted you to medicine? What are you most looking forward to in being a medical student and a doctor?

If you don't get into medicine, what are your plans?

Medical Education at a Glance, First Edition. Edited by Judy McKimm, Kirsty Forrest and Jill Thistlethwaite © 2017 John Wiley & Sons, Ltd. Published 2017 by John Wiley & Sons, Ltd.

Selection processes are used to recruit individuals into each of the various stages of education and training, and for subsequent jobs as a fully qualified professional. Whilst selection processes differ depending on the stage of training or career, some common features exist and an understanding of the purpose and format of these can help applicants perform better. Because places/posts are limited and competition is usually fairly fierce, universities, postgraduate training organisations and healthcare organisations need to put a series of hurdles in place with the aim of finding the best person for the job. Although selectors are looking to predict potential or future performance, this is difficult to do and so a range of instruments are used. Selection processes typically consider a series of essential and desirable criteria based around:

- Academic or professional qualifications – does the applicant meet the agreed level needed for the place/post?
- Skills or competencies – includes practical skills (e.g. surgical competence) as well as non-technical skills such as written and verbal communication or leadership
- Motivation, interest, enthusiasm for the place/post
- Aptitude for the role
- Views of other people who know the applicant, e.g. managers, referees, teachers.

In order to assess applicants against stated criteria, selection processes may involve written components, for example application form (including the 'open space' completed by applicants), essay, evidence of past performance or tests; practical components such as an Objective Structured Clinical Examination (OSCE) or simulation and evaluation of communication skills, for example interview, engagement in social events, group activities and presentation. For some senior posts, these activities may take place over a number of days so that the organisation can get feedback from and the opinion of a wide range of potential colleagues.

Interviews

Interviews are usually carried out face-to-face (or via video conference or telephone) with the applicant answering a series of structured questions from two or more people aimed at identifying their strengths, motivation, understanding of the organisation/post and how well they communicate. Sometimes applicants will be required to give a presentation, for example on what they see the challenges of the role. Although interviews have been criticised for being selective, subject to interviewer bias, unreliable and lacking in validity, they do give employers or recruiters opportunity to meet candidates and see them in action.

Selecting for professional attributes

It is relatively straightforward for organisations to be certain that applicants have the required academic and professional qualifications and that they are trained to a certain level (e.g. through graduation certificates or Royal College membership examinations). Aptitude tests, such as the MCAT (Medical College Admissions Test), UKCAT (UK Clinical Aptitude Test) or GAMSAT (Graduate Australian Medical Admissions Test), test for verbal or numerical ability and reasoning and have been shown to have predictive ability for future success in medical school (e.g. McManus et al., 2013).

The application form, interview, references and written tests can help provide some information, certainly enough to screen out those who do not meet threshold standards. However, in medicine and health care, it is vital that the organisations selecting individuals can be as assured as much as possible that they have the desired professional attributes. This is much harder to ascertain and predict. Of course, if someone has been subject to criminal proceedings, or disciplinary or fitness to practice procedures, then a red flag will be raised. But for the vast majority of applicants (particularly those applying to medical school) it is very challenging to select for professional attributes such as integrity, honesty, compassion, team-working or coping under pressure. In order to address this, new selection methods have been introduced, including psychometric tests and group activities. Two of the most widely used additional selection methods are described here.

Situational Judgement Tests

The Situational Judgement Test (SJT) is now used for selection to many medical schools and postgraduate training programmes. The SJT is a written multiple choice test in which candidates have to select which they think is the best response to a dilemma-based scenario. The aim of the SJT is to identify applicants who might lack elements of professional judgement (Patterson et al., 2016).

Multiple Mini Interviews

Multiple Mini Interviews (MMIs) have been used in selection for medicine for a number of years. Based on the design of the OSCE, MMIs require candidates to move around a series of 10–12 brief stations (e.g. 5–10 minutes) at which one or two interviewers ask questions based on previous experiences, defined situations or practical tests (Figure 9.2). Eva and Macala (2014) describe this situation in one station:

You are in your first year of medicine. In your PBL (problem-based learning) group of five students, you are encouraged to share your knowledge, teach each other, and contribute to the discussion. However, you notice that one of your colleagues is often quiet, shy and participates very little in the discussion. He also appears to do the minimum required work and his lack of participation is causing problems for the group. What would you do in this situation?

Eva and Macala, 2014, p. 607.

Although test content differs depending on the organisation and its goals, both the SJT and MMI provide a means of assessing a range of professional attributes, including coping with pressure; effective communication; learning and professional development; organisation and planning; patient focus; problem solving and decision making; self-awareness and insight and working effectively as part of a team. As such, they are moving in some way to better identify suitable and unsuitable individuals for medicine and for specific jobs.

10 Evaluation

Medical Education at a Glance, First Edition. Edited by Judy McKimm, Kirsty Forrest and Jill Thistlethwaite © 2017 John Wiley & Sons, Ltd. Published 2017 by John Wiley & Sons, Ltd.

Practice points

- Evaluation is used to drive change and improve quality
- Ideally it should focus on both process and outcomes
- Mixed methods are needed to gather rich data
- Changes made should be fed back to stakeholders

Box 10.1 Questions to consider when planning an evaluation

- What is the purpose of this evaluation?
- Who is it for?
- Are we planning to publish (consider ethics approval)?
- What data do we need?
- When will we collect it?
- How will we collect it?
- How will the data be analysed?
- Who will do the analysis?
- Is this a short-term or long-term evaluation or both?
- What will it cost?

Box 10.2 Questions to consider for outcomes evaluation

- What do we want the learners to learn?
- How will we know they have learned?
- How do we want the learners to change?
- How will we know they have changed?
- Will the learners behave differently after the intervention?
- How do we measure any change in behaviour?
- Were the learners satisfied?
- Were the educators satisfied?
- What could/should be improved next time?
- What is the longer-term impact?

Table 10.1 Outcomes-based evaluation

		What is measured?	Examples of methods
1	Learner reaction/ satisfaction	Learners' perceptions of their educational experiences; self assessment of change such as in skills, knowledge, confidence	Questionnaires, interviews, focus groups
2a	Modification of attitudes	Frequently used in the evaluation of interprofessional learning	Pre- and postlearning validated attitudinal surveys
2b	Acquisition of knowledge or skills	Learning in relation to previously defined learning outcomes or competencies	MCQs, extended matching pairs, OSCEs, simulations, simulated patient consultations
3	Change in behaviour or performance	Transfer of learning to the clinical setting	Work-based assessment, including direct observation, mini-CEX, multisource feedback
4a	Change in organisational practice	Rarely considered at the prequalification level; systems change at the postqualification training level	Audits, significant event analysis and follow-up, ethnographic studies, cost analyses
4b	Outcomes for patients or clients	Improvements in patient satisfaction, health outcomes	Patient satisfaction questionnaires, health indices, morbidity and mortality data

Abbrev: Mini-CEX, Mini-Clinical Exercise; MCQs, multiple choice questions; OSCE, Objective Structured Clinical Examination.

Source: adapted from Kirkpatrick and Kirkpatrick, 2006 and Barr *et al.*, 1999.

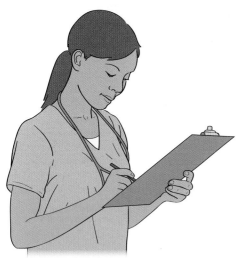

The purpose of evaluation

Educators undertake evaluation to find out the *value* of their programmes, sometimes (but not always) against external reference points – it is therefore a values-based, judgmental activity. Evaluation should be used to drive change, to improve the processes leading to learning and to ensure education is fit for purpose. Whilst evaluation and research may utilise similar methodologies and participant groups, educational research usually requires ethics approval and overt consent from participants, whereas evaluation does not. However, well-conceived, theoretically framed evaluations of educational innovations may still lead to publication and add to our discipline's evidence base. Note that in this chapter we are considering evaluation in relation to education delivery, as distinct from assessment of learners, which is sometimes referred to as evaluation, particularly in the US. Evaluation focuses on what is done or delivered (the programme), while assessment focuses on what learners have learned (the learners). Of course, assessment may be one component of an evaluation – we need to judge if and what learners learn.

An expert in this field, Michael Quinn Patton, defines evaluation as a 'systematic collection of information about the activities, characteristics and results of programs to make judgments about the program, improve or further develop program effectiveness, inform decisions about future programming, and/or increase understanding' (Patton, 2008, p. 39). In this statement, 'programme' may refer to many types of projects and innovations as well as education. In addition, though frequently omitted, evaluation should also consider cost and efficiency as well as outcomes (Rossi *et al.*, 2004).

Evaluation is mandatory in higher education institutions (HEIs) for quality assurance and may form part of an academic or clinician's annual performance review. Students are regularly asked to provide feedback on their teaching and opportunities for learning. Some students complain that there is, in fact, too much evaluation and that they are never informed of how their input is used.

As evaluation serves to measure the effectiveness of education, we need to define effectiveness. This may be whether learners have achieved defined learning outcomes but also whether they are satisfied with their overall experience at medical school or in training. The meaning of educational success may vary amongst stakeholders such as students, teachers, health professionals, patients, employers, accreditation bodies and policy makers. Therefore there is really no 'one size fits all' method of evaluation – it needs to be tailored to the evaluation question and the audience for the output. Short-term evaluation may be valuable for local use but longer-term impact studies are necessary for evidence of sustained learning and health services' improvement; such studies are rarely funded (Box 10.1).

Outcomes-based evaluation

The majority of the evaluation carried out in higher (tertiary) education is outcome or goals based – has the intervention achieved its stated goals? It is therefore obvious that the goals must be defined, made explicit, specific and clear, and also that they can be measured. Measurements usually occur at the end of the intervention. If a more detailed examination of change is required, learners may be compared before and after the intervention, or groups undergoing different programmes with similar learning outcomes may be compared (Box 10.2).

The Kirkpatrick Framework

A common framework used in health professional (and medical education) is that of Kirkpatrick (Kirkpatrick and Kirkpatrick, 2006), which was originally conceived in 1959 to evaluate training programmes in business and retail, with a major outcome being increase in sales revenue. In its original format, it is a four-tier model of educational outcomes with evidence being generated in relation to:

1 (Learners') reaction
2 Learning
3 Behaviour
4 Results.

The framework was subsequently adapted and expanded to six categories for the evaluation of interprofessional education (IPE) in 1999 (Barr *et al.*, 1999). The modified model has two outcomes under learning (level 2) and two under results (level 4) with a distinction between outcomes that relate to people and those that have an impact on health service delivery (Barr *et al.*, 2005); see Table 10.1. Kirkpatrick and Kirkpatrick (2006, p. 21) stipulated that the levels '…represent a sequence of ways to evaluate programs. Each level is important and has an impact on the next level. As you move from one level to the next, the process becomes more difficult and time-consuming, but it also provides more valuable information. None of the levels should be bypassed simply to get to the level that the trainer considers the most important.'

Most published evaluations concentrate on learner reaction with a combination of Likert scales and free-text comment boxes. Frequent items include student satisfaction, self-assessment of change in knowledge or confidence, and suggestions for changes to the intervention (Thistlethwaite *et al.*, 2015). Outcomes-based evaluation is important for programme development but focuses on 'does this work' rather than 'how and why does it work/not work', the latter requiring a process approach. Notable criticisms of the Kirkpatrick method include that of Yardley and Dornan (2012) who conclude that the framework is unsuitable for other than relatively simple educational designs, not the complexity of health professions' education.

Process evaluation

Outcomes-based evaluation may show that 70% of students passed an assessment following an innovative way of learning. While this shows the method was effective in enhancing the knowledge or skills of the majority of students, educators may want to know why nearly one-third of the cohort 'failed'. To evaluate a programme in these terms, we need to look at the process of learning and teaching, and this will require a mixed methods approach (quantitative and qualitative). Process evaluation is usually more time-consuming and requires an in-depth analysis of data. It may involve observation of learners and facilitators during formal sessions, interviews or focus groups with learners to explore engagement or why sessions have been rated poorly, and interviews with staff to probe into how examination marks are awarded.

Realist evaluation is a specific form of process evaluation that considers 'What works for whom and in what contexts?' (Pawson and Tilley, 1997). It acknowledges the complexity inherent in education and its lack of a linear causation in terms of inputs and outcomes. The method has been recommended for use in medical education (Wong *et al.*, 2012) but is less likely to be used for day-to-day evaluation.

11 Educational leadership

Figure 11.1 Leadership in threes. Source: McKimm et al., 2016.

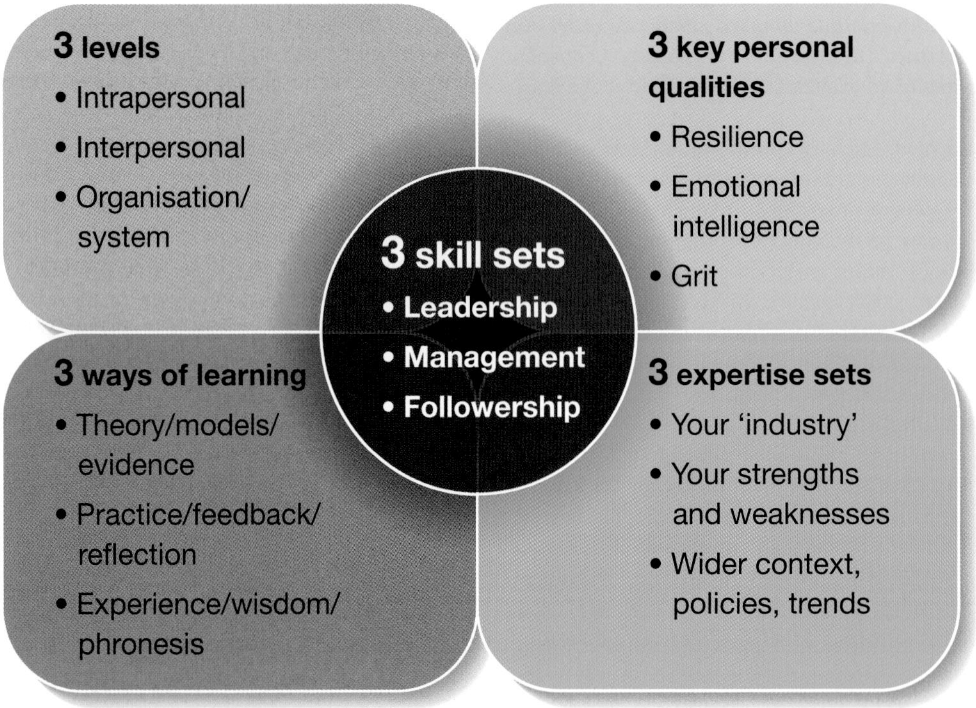

3 levels
- Intrapersonal
- Interpersonal
- Organisation/ system

3 key personal qualities
- Resilience
- Emotional intelligence
- Grit

3 skill sets
- Leadership
- Management
- Followership

3 ways of learning
- Theory/models/ evidence
- Practice/feedback/ reflection
- Experience/wisdom/ phronesis

3 expertise sets
- Your 'industry'
- Your strengths and weaknesses
- Wider context, policies, trends

Figure 11.2 The leadership triad

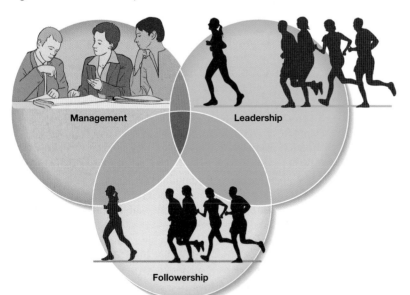

Management

Leadership

Followership

Box 11.1 The leadership 'triad' in practice

You are running an Objective Structured Clinical Examination (OSCE) for 300 medical students.

- What management skills do you use to ensure you get everything done properly?
- If a crisis occurs (three examiners don't turn up or one of the students faints at station 3), you might need leadership or followership skills as well?
- What skills will you need to use?

Medical Education at a Glance, First Edition. Edited by Judy McKimm, Kirsty Forrest and Jill Thistlethwaite © 2017 John Wiley & Sons, Ltd. Published 2017 by John Wiley & Sons, Ltd.

Leadership can be defined as 'a process whereby an individual influences a group of individuals to achieve a common goal' (Northouse, 2010, p. 3). On a day to day basis, medical educational leadership involves working with learners and staff from universities and healthcare organisations with the aim of educating and training doctors effectively and efficiently. Leadership involves decision making, team leadership, self-management and high-level communication skills. Drawing widely from the literature and our own research, the leadership in threes model (Figure 11.1) provides a way of conceptualising a set of interrelated concepts and the essentials of effective leadership (McKimm *et al.,* 2016).

Leadership approaches

The leadership literature is vast, but the main approaches to understanding leadership can be summarised as follows:
- **Trait theories** – focussing on personality traits and a list of qualities (e.g. integrity, charisma, approachability, concern).
- **Style theories** – how the leader behaves in different situations (e.g. authoritative, consultative), takes account that leadership can be modified and learned.
- **Transactional and transformational** – transactional relates to management and involves exchange of effort for reward (e.g. you work for an employer and you get paid). Transformational leadership is about leaders inspiring and motivating others towards higher order goals or values. Whilst this is appealing in education, the realities of managed systems with targets and performance measures can lead to cynicism.
- **Collaborative, shared, distributed and collective leadership** – these approaches look at leadership at all levels of an organisation and consider that it is only by working together that real change and improvement will be made.
- **Adaptive leadership** – is about working in complex, uncertain systems and times and adapting ways of working to develop solutions to new or 'wicked' problems.
- **Eco-leadership, value-led, servant and moral leadership** – all involve 'making a difference' through engaging with the moral purpose and values of organisations, and looking to environmental and societal sustainability.
- **Inclusive and person-centred leadership** – embrace diversity and have the needs of people at their heart.

Three skills sets

Figures 11.1 and 11.2 set out three interlinked skills sets: the 'leadership triad' (McKimm and O'Sullivan, 2016). Management is about planning, providing stability and order (doing things right) whereas leadership is about change, setting direction and adaptability (doing the right thing). Organisations, teams or situations need both leadership and management in varying amounts depending on the situation or context. Of course, we do not lead all the time and being able to be a good follower (who is supportive, active, questioning and helpful) is important to ensure groups, teams and organisations function smoothly. The concept of 'little 'l' leadership' (Kelley, 1988; Bohmer, 2010) is helpful for taking small steps into leadership through managing a project, leading an initiative or new role and can help people see where their role fits in the curriculum or organisation.

Three levels

Leadership skills, models and theories (and your own development) can be thought of in terms of three overlapping categories (Swanwick and McKimm, 2014):

Intrapersonal – focussing on the personal qualities or personality of the leader; involves getting to know yourself and developing self-insight, understanding your strengths and weaknesses and how you respond under pressure.

Interpersonal – relating to the interaction of the leader with others; working in teams, with other health workers, patients and families. How do others see you?

Organisational/system wide – leadership in relation to the organisation or system; involves learning about and understanding the wider health system, your organisation, politics and processes and how change and improvement may be managed.

Three expertise sets

Leaders need to have credibility, and we suggest this can be developed in three ways. Firstly, by understanding your industry – for us this is medical education. As 'educationalists', leaders need to understand how education systems, structures, funding and programmes work and possess a theoretical educational knowledge. Secondly, understanding the wider sociocultural, political and economic context will help you keep abreast of trends and policies that might affect the education you provide and help you identify and seize opportunities. Becoming an expert in your area, project or initiative helps to build credibility, particularly when your power and influence is relatively low because of position in the organisation and professional hierarchies (Till *et al.,* 2014). Thirdly, understanding your strengths and weaknesses helps you to build effective teams and structure your leadership development.

Three key personal qualities

The leadership literature identifies a plethora of personal qualities leaders should have (including integrity, humility and charisma), and also notes the harmful effect *toxic* or *destructive* leadership has. However, three qualities encompass the majority of the qualities of successful leaders: resilience, emotional intelligence and grit. Resilience is the ability to bounce back from adversity or challenge. Emotional intelligence (EI) comprises a combination of self-awareness, empathy, social skills, self-motivation and self-regulation (Goleman, 2000). Grit is a combination of resilience, passion, hard work, perseverance, determination and direction (Duckworth, 2016). To be 'gritty' you have to have a deep interest in what you're doing; take opportunities to practice skills and show self-discipline; cultivate a conviction and purpose about your work (it has to matter); and have hope and confidence that you can *do* leadership as well as *be* a leader.

Three ways of learning

Many formal opportunities exist for medical educators to learn leadership through short courses, workshops and longer, award bearing programmes. Such 'horizontal leadership' (Petrie, 2014) provide an evidence base (in terms of theories, concept, models and tools) about what leadership is, how it works and ways of approaching situations or tasks. However, it is only through practice, obtaining constructive feedback and reflection that you will learn for yourself how to lead, follow and manage effectively. This involves 'vertical leadership': meeting challenges (heat experiences); sense-making of the experience (through reflection and conversation) and being open to colliding perspectives about what is going on (Petrie, 2014). Learning leadership is therefore a lifelong endeavour; good leaders have learned from their experiences and gained a practical wisdom (phronesis) about how to behave and function in different situations.

12 International perspectives

Practice points

- Medical education is now a global enterprise with blurred boundaries between the medical education on offer in different countries
- Learners need to be prepared to work internationally as well as locally
- The decision to move to another country needs careful consideration about a number of personal and professional aspects

Box 12.1 Questions about personal and professional issues when considering an academic position abroad

Personal issues

- Will I need to learn another language?
- Am I sufficiently adaptable and tolerant of cultural or religious practices that may challenge my ethical and professional values?
- Where can I find out what it is like to work in such a context?
- Do I travel alone or do I bring my family? What are the pros and cons?
- Is it safe to be a single female or appropriate to be a single male?
- Are there health risks?
- What are the tax implications back in my home country?

Professional issues

- What does this position mean in terms of my career trajectory?
- Does my medical qualification allow me to practice clinically?
- Am I required to maintain my medical certification?

Box 12.2 Key principles underpinning electives

Planning stages: Questions

- What is the purpose of the elective?
- What resources are available at the facility?
- What health risks might I encounter?
- What preventative measures are needed?
- What personal risks might I encounter?
- What ethical standards should I expect?
- What cultural and/or religious practices should I be aware of?
- How do I communicate with health care workers and the patients?
- Have I attended the pre-departure briefing?
- Are my clinical skills honed?

During the elective: Questions

- Am I working within my scope of practice?
- What do I do if there is an expectation that I undertake a procedure that I have not previously done?
- What do I do if I see another student engaging in unethical behaviour?

Returning from an elective: Questions

- What do I need to do on my return?

Figure 12.1 Model depicting the development of an international medical educator. Source: McLean *et al.*, 2014. Reproduced with permission of Taylor & Francis.

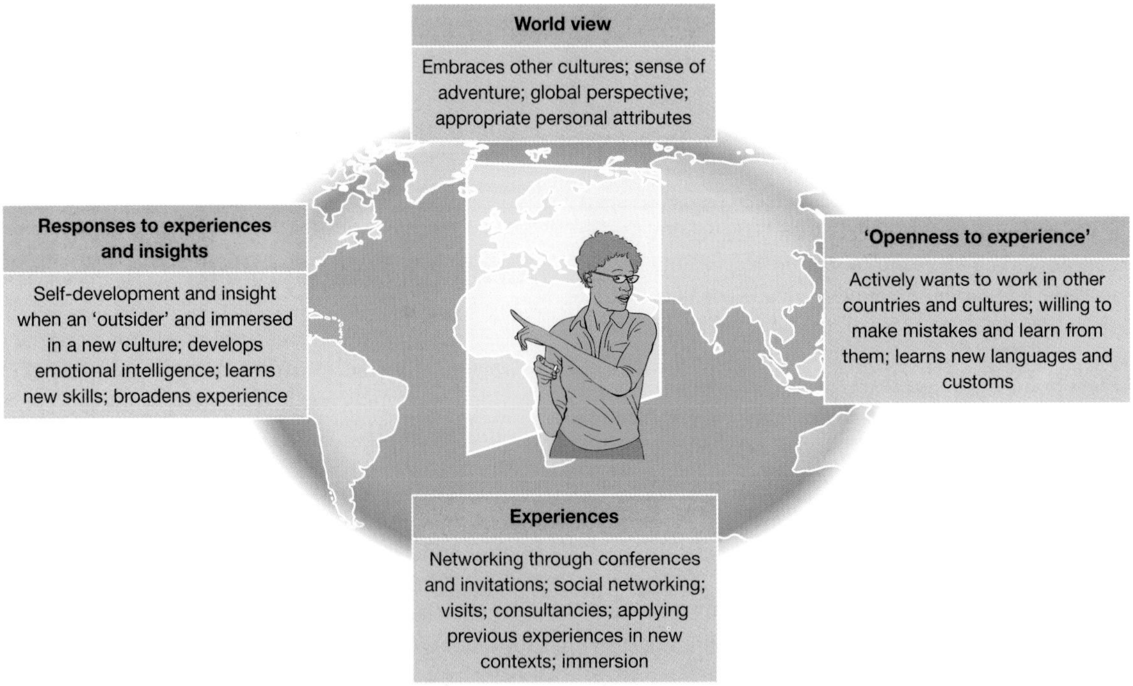

World view

Embraces other cultures; sense of adventure; global perspective; appropriate personal attributes

Responses to experiences and insights

Self-development and insight when an 'outsider' and immersed in a new culture; develops emotional intelligence; learns new skills; broadens experience

'Openness to experience'

Actively wants to work in other countries and cultures; willing to make mistakes and learn from them; learns new languages and customs

Experiences

Networking through conferences and invitations; social networking; visits; consultancies; applying previous experiences in new contexts; immersion

We live in a global world, a world in which digital and communication technologies allow us to connect instantly with family, friends and colleagues across numerous times zones and in far flung corners of the globe. It is also a world in which political and economic unions and affordable air travel have facilitated the ease with which individuals can cross national borders. It is, however, also a world in which higher education is now a commodity and a market-driven business. Medical education is no exception, with the number of available places far exceeding prospective applicants, sometimes in the order of 10-12-fold. This demand has resulted in many traditional universities in Europe, North America and Australia actively recruiting full fee-paying international students while other institutions have established offshore campuses in emerging economies such as the Middle East, Asia and the Caribbean.

International learners, doctors and teachers

The past decade has seen a changing medical student and medical graduate profile. For students and practising doctors studying and working in new countries and cultures, many challenges are involved including language, social, financial and professional implications (McKimm and Wilkinson, 2015).

Medical educators have also been on the move. Often spurred by a desire to experience different cultural and academic contexts, medical educators choose to work abroad for both personal (e.g. family, altruism, financial) and professional reasons (e.g. research, professional development) (McLean *et al.,* 2014). With this international status come pros and cons for both the educator and the employing institution. On the positive side, the institution can use the educator's expertise to improve or develop programmes while students would be enriched through exposure to different worldviews. The educator too learns different ways of doing and seeing things.

The decision to move countries and cultures should, however, not be taken lightly by anyone. The personal and professional implications should be well researched, particularly if the cultural context is far removed from one's own. While such a move often has language implications, not only for the individual but also for their family, the organisational culture may also be challenging in terms of academic autonomy. Box 12.1 provides a series of questions and answers for an individual considering becoming an international medical educator (which also apply to doctors and learners) whilst Figure 12.1 provides a model depicting the evolution of (i.e. *becoming* and *being*) an international medical educator. The model encompasses one's worldview, openness to experiences, the actual experiences, reflection on the new and sometimes challenging immersion in a new culture and the insight gained.

Towards transnational medical education

In his 2006 article on the future directions of medical education in a rapidly globalising world, Harden envisaged a shift from a context in which both the teacher and the students were local to a transnational scenario in which internationalisation is embedded within a curriculum that involves collaboration between a number of schools in different countries. While this is still an emerging scenario, increasingly in medical education circles we can add the word 'international' to our descriptions of medical students, medical educators and to the curriculum.

Internationalisation of the curriculum

With students travelling to other countries or regions to study medicine and then returning to their home countries to practice, the curriculum must reflect this. A common adage in medical education circles today is 'think globally, act locally', meaning that a medical programme should produce graduates able to practice anywhere in the world, but who can also adapt to meet local needs. Several models exist, ranging from one in which students complete part of their training abroad and then complete their degree in their home country, to one in which the content has a more global focus and students undertake both local and international electives to develop their broad scope of practice.

Global health and international electives and social accountability

Global health and international health electives are two hot topics in medical education, largely because of another imperative – *social accountability*. To meet the challenges of the twenty-first century, a Global Consensus on Social Accountability of Medical Schools, has identified ten strategic directions for medical schools to become socially accountable to improve society's current and future health needs and challenges (Figure 12.2). These include reorienting education, research and service priorities, strengthening governance and partnerships with stakeholders and by using evaluation and accreditation to assess performance and impact.

Although many well established medical schools now have formal partnerships and exchanges with institutions in developing countries to ensure mutual benefits and safe practice, this is not always the case. Some medical schools expect but do not arrange students' international electives, leaving students to arrange their electives, which may mean paying a private company. Whatever the circumstances, any elective in which there is a potential power differential between students and the patients should be underpinned by fundamental humanitarian principles.

Figure 12.2 Global consensus on social accountability: ten areas for action. Source: http://healthsocialaccountability.sites.olt.ubc.ca/files/2011/06/11-06-07-GCSA-English-pdf-style.pdf (accessed Sept. 2016). Reproduced with permission of Global Consensus on Social Accountability.

Global Consensus for Social Accountability
OF MEDICAL SCHOOLS

Area 1	Anticipating society's health needs
Area 2	Partnering the health system and other stakeholders
Area 3	Adapting to the changing role of doctors and other health professionals
Area 4	Fostering outcome-based education
Area 5	Creating responsive and responsible governance of the medical school
Area 6	Refining the scope of standards for education, research and service delivery
Area 7	Supporting continous quality improvement in education, research and service delivery
Area 8	Establishing mandated mechanisms for accreditation
Area 9	Balancing global principles with context specificity
Area 10	Defining the role of society

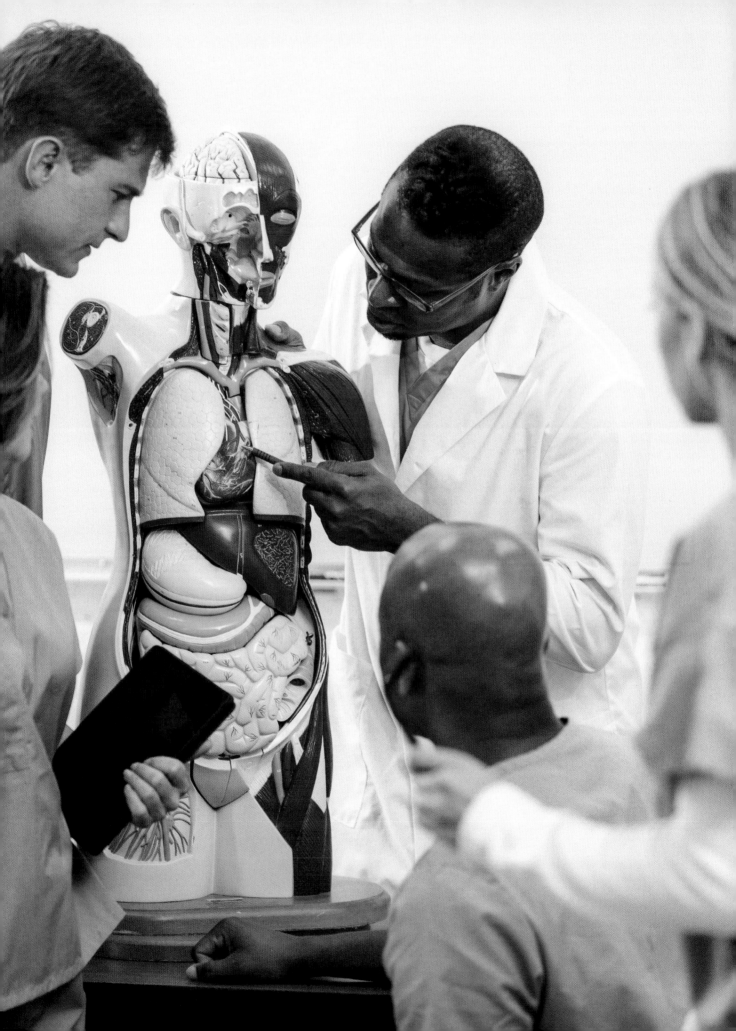

Medical education in practice

Part 2

Chapters

13 Large group teaching: planning and design

Practice points

- Being able to work with large groups confidently and effectively is essential for many educators
- Lecturing can be made more interesting and interactive with the use of specific techniques
- Lectures are inappropriate for skills acquisition and in-depth discussion
- Planning the session and practising presentations are vital

Figure 13.1 Lecture theatre

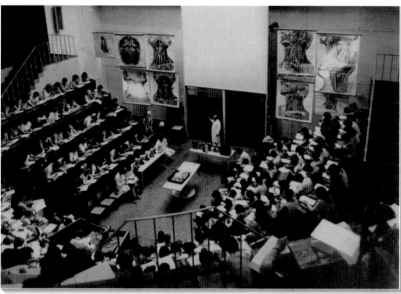

Source: Bundesarchiv, Bild 183-Z0622-007/Grubitzsch (geb. Raphael), Waltraud,
https://commons.wikimedia.org/wiki/File:Bundesarchiv_Bild_183-Z0622-007,_Leipzig,_Universität,_Hörsaal,_Anatomievorlesung.jpg
Used under CC-BY-SA 3.0 https://creativecommons.org/licenses/by-sa/3.0/

Figure 13.2 A bad power point slide

> **Background**
>
> - Avoid backgrounds that are distracting or difficult to read from
> - Always be consistent with the background that you use

Figure 13.3 Example lesson plan. Source: *Essential Guide to Generic Skills.* Copyright © 2006 Nicola Cooper, Kirsty Forrest and Paul Cramp. Published by Blackwell Publishing Ltd. Reproduced with permission of Kirsty Forrest.

Lecture: Physiology and pharmacology of pain
Aims: Understanding the physiology and pharmacological treatment of pain

Timing (min)	Teacher activity	Student activity	Resources
5	Introduction Definition Assessment	Listening	PowerPoint
10	Introduce the stickman and ask the students in buzz groups to draw the pain pathways on it	Buzz groups	Paper stick man
5	Get back answers from the groups	One student at the front filling in flip chart, the others providing the answers	Flip chart
15	The introduction of analgesic drugs	Listening	PowerPoint
10	On the paper stickman draw were the analgesic drugs work	Buzz groups	Paper stickman
5	Get back answers from the groups	One student at the front filling in flip chart, the others providing the answers	Flip chart
5	Summary Questions	Questions	Handout Filled in stickman Analgesic ladder

Giving lectures to large groups of students has been a traditional way of teaching for hundreds of years (Figure 13.1). With shifts in learning approaches and the more widespread use of online learning, the use of lectures as a primary means of teaching has fallen out of favour. This quote is often used to highlight the dissatisfaction:

A lecture: the process by which the notes of the professor become the notes of the student without ever passing through the mind of either.

Miller, 1927, p. 120.

However, lectures are still effective in:
• Teaching large groups economically. The ratio of teacher to student can be as much as 1 : 300 or even more now with podcasts and WebEx facilities
• Providing core knowledge, delivery of course content, principles, facts, terminology and concepts
• Demonstrating enthusiasm of teachers for their subject
• Directing and scaffolding learning.
    The limitations of lectures include:
• Inadequate for skills teaching
• Not necessarily good for abstract or complex issues, which need discussion
• Hard to integrate with other connected sessions
• Make significant demands on the attention span of an audience.

Planning a lecture

When planning any teaching episode you must consider:

1 The environment

You are responsible for ensuring that the lighting, temperature, acoustics and seating are all conducive to learning. Even before you start to plan the educational content of a lecture, there are important logistics to consider: the venue, how many students will be there, the acoustics and lighting and what audio-visual equipment is provided. You should try to visit the lecture theatre beforehand to familiarise yourself with the equipment.

2 The set

Before any teaching episode, including lectures, you should ask three questions: Who am I teaching? (e.g. medical students, nursing staff or residents); What do they already know? (e.g. is this teaching part of a course); What do they want me to teach? (i.e. what are the aims and objectives of this session?). All teaching episodes should start with an outline or list of objectives. If you do not tell the learner the aims and objectives of the session they will find it hard to follow the whole process. For the learner, this is like solving a jigsaw puzzle without seeing the picture.

3 The dialogue or delivery of the lecture.

The next step is to deliver information. Aristotle is quoted as saying: 'tell your audience what you are going to tell them, tell them, and then tell them what you just told them' (Gross and Walzer, 2000). Whilst this is a good basic structure, there are many other ways of doing this. One can look at things systematically, tell a story or state a problem and provide an answer. There is more about delivery in Chapter 14.

4 Closure – summary and questions.

At the end you should provide a summary of what you have said and any follow-up activities or links to other parts of the programme.

Presentations

Most lecturers now use PowerPoint or similar computer-based delivery method to deliver their lectures. However, there are pitfalls and limitations to using these and presentations are definitely a case of 'less is more'. Using PowerPoint can provide a useful way of planning your lecture and ensuring there is a 'story' that puts over your key messages. The slides should provide a basis for or summary of what you say, do not cram every word onto the slides and then read the slides. This is not what a lecture is all about. Too many pictures, fancy PowerPoint slide transitions, sound effects and use of humour can also detract from the main message. Rehearse your presentation for timekeeping and sense making.

Always be prepared for the fact that the technology might go wrong. Check in advance what type of computer is being used for compatibility between systems and whether you need to have the presentation on a USB port or it will be centrally loaded. For really high-stakes presentations (e.g. interview or conference keynote) if appropriate, it is wise to have your set of slides on back-up handouts as well. If travelling, when things might get lost, post your presentation to your webmail account before setting off and check the presentation on the computer you'll be using, as versions vary and fonts, backgrounds etc. can become distorted.

PowerPoint tips (see also Figure 13.2):
• Only use contrasting colours, for example white text on a dark blue background or black text on a white background
• Use no more than two colours per slide
• Do not use capital letters – they are difficult to read
• Plan your talk using roughly 1 minute per slide
• Use large font (e.g. 24–32 point), preferably PC friendly such as Ariel, Tahoma or Verdana
• There should be no more than six bullet points per slide
• Avoid overuse of cute Clipart or cartoons
• Make sure you cite source or get permissions for visuals – best to use *Creative Commons* for open source images.

Lecture planning

A useful exercise for any educational episode is to plan it on paper as a lesson plan. Your lesson plan should include the aims and objectives, timings for each section of the lecture and which equipment you will be using for that section, see Chapter 7 and Figure 13.3 for example lesson plans.

Although many lecturers do not like giving out handouts at the start of a lecture, students tend to prefer them. Appropriate handouts provide:
• An outline of the lecture to help learners follow it more easily and allow them to concentrate on listening and processing the information as they hear it, instead of concentrating on transcribing every word. Later, the outline will help them review their notes and reflect on the content of the lecture
• Essential diagrams so learners are listening and engaging, not drawing pictures
• Materials that learners may find difficult or impossible to obtain elsewhere
• Questions and tasks that will encourage learners to reflect on their learning
• Gaps / spaces so that learners can fill in text or complete
• A supplementary reading list.

14 Large group teaching: delivery

Figure 14.1 Lectures should be stimulating

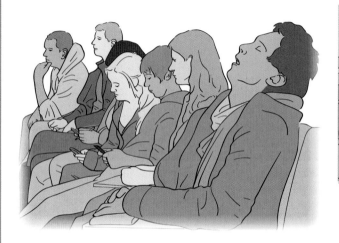

Figure 14.2 Keep focus on the audience

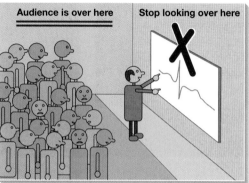

Figure 14.3 Student learning and interactivity. Source: *Essential Guide to Generic Skills.* Copyright © 2006 Nicola Cooper, Kirsty Forrest and Paul Cramp. Published by Blackwell Publishing Ltd. Reproduced with permission of Kirsty Forrest.

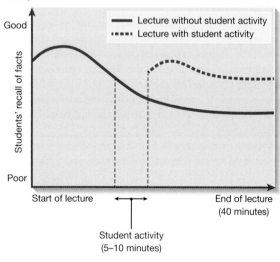

Figure 14.4 Learning pyramid. Source: The National Training Laboratories Institute (Bethel, Maine).

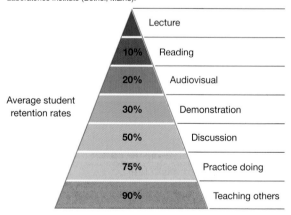

Effective lecturing is more a matter of skill than charisma, although there are some techniques that can help to make your lectures more enjoyable for those in the audience (Figure 14.1). Research about what students liked in lectures (Ramsden, 1992) shows that they appreciate:

• Material pitched at the right level
• Clear structure
• Appropriate pace
• Enthusiasm
• Ability to provide good explanations
• Variety and interactivity.

Practice makes perfect

How we put our message across is as important as what we have to say. There are three elements to face to face communication, known as the '7% (words) 38% (tone of voice) 55% (body language) rule' (Mehrabian, 1971). These figures were derived from experiments dealing with communication of feelings and attitudes and convey the importance of non-verbal communication. Practice looking confident and smiling at the audience. Someone will always smile back even if the audience are complete strangers (try this, it really does work) and this will help you relax and look more confident.

Only very experienced lecturers can operate without a script. Most people need to have their talk written out in front of them which they can refer to as they go along. Rehearsal is important. Ask a colleague if they will listen to you practice. Memorise the first 30 seconds of your presentation so as not to look down at your prompts too early. Speak so slowly that it feels strange to you. We all speak faster than we should, partly because of nerves, and sometimes due to enthusiasm. If your presentation requires a microphone, use it, rather than eyeing it suspiciously or moving around so that the volume of your voice changes. Giving a good presentation requires acting skills. Dress conservatively, smartly and comfortably. People should not be distracted by what you are wearing.

Top tips for body language:
• Stand still with both feet apart and one foot slightly forward.
• Use a lectern for security and notes.
• Put your arms by your sides or on the lectern apart from the occasional gesture.
• Face the audience (see Figure 14.2).
• Make eye contact with all areas of the room.
• Smile, be enthusiastic and natural.
• Know your bad habits, for example covering your mouth when speaking, making funny faces, scratching your nose, nervous cough or jangling coins in your pocket.

Scaffolding and signposting

It is important that your lecture appears coherent and logical to your audience. Signal stages of your structure by using the following.

Signposts: statements that indicate the structure and direction of an explanation (e.g. 'I want to deal briefly with... First, I will outline... Next, we shall look into these points in greater detail...').

Frames: statements that signal the beginning and the end of a section (e.g. 'So that ends my discussion of... And now, let us look at...'). Framing statements are particularly important in complex explanations that may involve topics and subtopics.

Foci: direct attention to key points by emphasis, repetition and through the use of statements that highlight key points (e.g. 'So the main point is...', 'The key issue here is...', 'This brings us to the crucial factor...').

Links: words, phrases or statements that link one part of an explanation to another (e.g. 'But while this may be the solution, it may lead to several complications and objections not directly related to it').

Summaries: these serve to remind students of the essential points and to link topics and themes that may have been separately discussed. Summarising provides an opportunity to compare and contrast, point to similarities and differences, advantages and disadvantages, etc.

How to introduce interactivity

Delivering a lecture can easily fall into the mode of transmission, passive, linear, information giving and teacher focussed. Research on lectures shows that the attention of students is highest for the first 10 minutes, then quickly falls before rising slightly before the end (Stuart and Rutherford, 1978). If a change in delivery or interactivity is introduced, attention rises again but never quite reaches the initial peak. Figure 14.3 illustrates this.

Depending on the length of the talk and the audience, the best lectures are more active, non-linear and student focussed, to increase attention and retention. Giving good lectures is not easy but does get better with practice. For experienced lecturers, interactivity can feel less controlled than the traditional way of reading out slides to a passive group. However, we have to remember that the point of a lecture is so that people can learn (Figure 14.4).

There are many ways to introduce interactivity to a lecture:
• Divide students into buzz groups, for example two students turn around to speak with the two students behind them. Ask the groups to address a question or problem on the screen. If the groups feed back, there is 'safety in numbers' so no one feels intimidated.
• Put up a question in the middle of the presentation that needs working out. For example, in a lecture on local anaesthesia ask students to work out doses for theoretical patients.
• Ask for answers to multiple choice questions (MCQs) on the screen by a show of hands or electronic voting system. This helps to establish whether students have understood the teaching so far.
• Change the media you are using. Move from PowerPoint to a flip chart or video.
• Build exercises into your handouts.

Sometimes large groups are not the best forum for questions as students may feel intimidated to speak up. Ways around this include saying that you will stay behind at the end to take questions; asking for written questions to be put on post-it notes or on a board during a break; using Twitter or text-based questions during the lecture. This enables you to select particular questions to address, especially if a number of students haven't understood something.

15 Small group teaching: planning and design

Table 15.1 Advantages and disadvantages of small group teaching

Advantages of small group teaching include:	Disadvantages of small group teaching include:
• Active participation	• Weak students may become discouraged
• Develops independence and maturity	• Bright students may become bored
• Facilitators can check students' understanding of subjects	• Some discussions may be irrelevant
• Learners can think critically and systematically	• Different opinions may lead to arguments
• Easier to deal with difficult subject matter	• Talkers can monopolise time and attention
• Fosters the ability to work in teams	• The tutor gives a lecture rather than facilitates
• Instant feedback can be given	• The tutor takes over and leads the discussion
• Students can ask questions that they feel unable to ask in lectures	• Lack of interaction from some students
• Students can learn from each other	• Lack of preparation by students
• Learning can be more student centred	• Students have nowhere to 'hide'
• It is a good place for tutors to role model attitudes	• Logistics – it requires more tutor time, more rooms and resources

Figure 15.1 Examples of small-group teaching

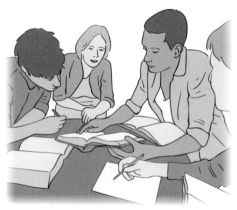
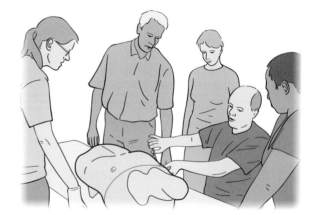
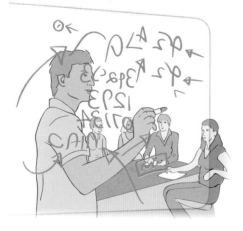

Medical Education at a Glance, First Edition. Edited by Judy McKimm, Kirsty Forrest and Jill Thistlethwaite © 2017 John Wiley & Sons, Ltd. Published 2017 by John Wiley & Sons, Ltd.

Healthcare professionals work in clinical small groups or teams in theatre, on the ward, in outpatients and in general practice. Generally, the acceptable size of a small group for teaching purposes is somewhere between five and 12 people. With fewer or more people than this, the ways in which the members of the group interact makes the small group function differently. Therefore, for the rest of this chapter, these numbers will form the working definition of a small group.

A variety of small group sessions exist: seminars, problem or case-based learning (see Chapter 31), tutorials, closed discussions, break out groups, open discussions, clinical skills sessions and workshops. With the rise of flipped classrooms, where the learning (often online) takes place independently prior to a group session, teachers need to be able to work in small group learning settings as well as lecture theatres or other venues. Have you been to a small group teaching session only to experience a lecture? In a small group, the teacher's role is to facilitate learning and understanding through discussion as well as imparting information. Small group teaching also requires active participation and collaboration by all present and often the production or completion of a task.

Why small group teaching?

Small group teaching is a way of 'teaching' that is facilitative, and more discursive than a lecture, leading to a broader (and hopefully deeper) learning episode. Small group teaching works well for parts of the curriculum that require synthesis and evaluation of knowledge and where students can discuss their understanding of concepts. Small group teaching also helps to foster generic skills that are very relevant to medicine: communication, leadership and co-operation. Another benefit of small group teaching is socialisation. Some students like to know how they are doing compared with others. There is nothing as good as finding out that you are not stupid and the rest of the class has been struggling to understand a concept as well. Table 15.1 lists the advantages and disadvantages to the learner of small group teaching.

Planning

Small group work is not appropriate for all of your learners' needs but by choosing the right topics and laying appropriate foundations, learners can get a great deal from them. A number of issues need to be considered when planning a small group session. In common with all teaching, you need to define the content and learning outcomes you wish to achieve. For small group teaching, you also need to consider the following aspects.

Group characteristics

Discussion groups are rarely successful with more than 12 participants and, depending on the nature of the task, six to eight might be more appropriate. If numbers exceed 12, formation of subgroups and splintering tends to happen so the group becomes less coherent. Knowing your group is important, including whether the group knows one other socially, academically or clinically as these dynamics will affect how a session will run. There may be varying levels of knowledge within a group; this will also affect the group dynamic and how comfortable people feel in contributing. The aim is to pitch the session at the right level so as to engage all whilst not confusing or boring others.

Interpersonal issues

The role of the group facilitator is to listen more than talk. After an initial statement, the facilitator should, through subtle use of body language and a particular approach to asking questions, allow the conversation to develop among the students, having them speaking to one another rather than directing everything to the facilitator. This stops the facilitator from having a judicial role, which is something that can be observed in adult education settings where sessions become, 'Emotional battlegrounds with members vying for recognition and affirmation from each other and from the discussion leader.' (Brookfield, 1993, p. 24). This is the socioemotional component of the learning environment and, unless it is well handled, can interfere with effective learning for many group members. More significant, however, is the nature of the interactions that are expected among the group.

Constraints of your environment

Clearly, you need sufficient space to seat everyone comfortably. If you are given a very large space, it is preferable to use a corner and, if possible, use lighting to help close down the surplus areas. People do not like to find themselves in the centre of large well-lit spaces as it makes them feel overlooked. It is not impossible that you might find yourself in a lecture theatre with fixed, possibly tiered seating. In these circumstances it is still possible to put together a group of about six to eight in a degree of comfort. Don't be afraid to change room layouts to suit your needs if possible. In general, the layout for a discussion group is more democratic than for a lecture to encourage participation. Apart from the size of the group it is more likely to encourage closer proximity and mutual eye contact.

Time frame

Many first-time facilitators underestimate the amount of time a session can take and do not take into account the actual discussion time, which by its nature is not predictable. They also try to include too much in one session, so taking time to plan and clarify expectations is important.

Ground rules

Setting ground rules for the group from the outset can often help define acceptable behaviours within a group. Ground rules are best set by the learners themselves. Examples might include: being on time (including the facilitator), maintaining confidentiality, not interrupting when someone is talking, switching phones to silent and respecting others' opinions, even though you might disagree with them.

16 Small group teaching: delivery

Practice points

- Small group facilitation needs good planning and use of various techniques to manage group dynamics and potentially disruptive behaviours
- Closed discussions are facilitator controlled throughout and suitable for more knowledge-based interactions
- Open discussions are useful for ethical or '*softer*' issues to encourage debate and learning from one another

Table 16.1 Responding to behaviours

Behaviour	Response
Asking for confirmation about the nature of the task	Making a clear and unambiguous statement in your opening comment but having it written up on a screen or flip chart can help
Asking for clarification	Saying something like 'As you see it'
Checking for affirmation (from facilitator and other group members)	Initiating the discussion, saying something like 'Tell us what you think'
Seeking approval	Saying something like 'What do others think?'
Talking off task	Inviting a direct response from the talker
Telling jokes	Acknowledging, laughing (if funny) and moving on: 'So …' to other side of circle
Describing work title/practices	Saying 'Tell us how […] fits with your experience'
Complaining about:	
the task	Ignoring
aspects of the environment	Asking the group 'Are you warm/cool enough?' and making environmental adjustments if appropriate
the programme	Ignoring
the facilitator	Ignoring
Giving way to dominant members	Asking for comments
Off-task fascination	Summarising and redirecting
Argumentative behaviour/personal attacks on other group member	Closing down the argumentative person

Source: Mike Davis, Kirsty Forrest. *How to Teach Continuing Medical Education*, 2008. BMJ Books. Reproduced with permission of Kirsty Forrest.

Figure 16.1 Seating arrangements. Source: McKimm and Morris, 2014.

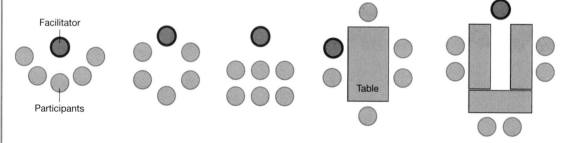

Table 16.2 Comparison of how different group sessions work

	Closed discussion	Workshop	Open discussion
Question and answers	Through the facilitator	Of one another	Of one another
Nature of dialogue	Closed questions to identified individuals	Open questions after initial direction	Open questions after initial direction
Arrangement of chairs	Horseshoe	Depends on content of workshop	Circle
Equipment	A/V	A/V clinical equipment	None
Role of facilitator	Steering the direction of discussion and providing a summary	Introduction, redirection, error correction and summary	Introduction, redirection and summary
Subject matter	Known answer to problem, e.g. 'causes of…'	Mainly known but applying known knowledge to new cases/contexts, e.g. looking at ECGs, skills teaching	Not necessarily any correct answers, e.g. ethical discussions

Medical Education at a Glance, First Edition. Edited by Judy McKimm, Kirsty Forrest and Jill Thistlethwaite © 2017 John Wiley & Sons, Ltd. Published 2017 by John Wiley & Sons, Ltd.

Facilitating small groups can be very rewarding and is a good way of getting to know your learners in more depth. However, all groups have to learn how to function together and in medical education, the facilitator is often (but not always) the group leader who needs to pay attention to this. Johnson and Johnson (Johnson and Johnson, 1987, cited in Jacques, 2010) suggest the following seven-stage model of group development: (1) Defining and structuring procedures; (2) Conforming to procedures and getting acquainted; (3) Recognising mutuality and building trust; (4) Rebelling and differentiating; (5) Committing to and taking ownership for the goals, procedures and other members; (6) Functioning maturely and productively; (7) Terminating.

Managing small groups requires a facilitator who might function in different ways:

- Chairperson – task centred (closed discussion)
- Facilitator – process centred (open discussion)
- Instructor – skill station
- Participant – no leader
- Devil's advocate – offers counter arguments
- Agitator – dislikes comfortable discussion, is provocative.

While the first three functions work well, it is best to avoid the last three functions as the group can get out of control and people can become uncomfortable or start acting out. These are learning groups, so the purpose is to facilitate learning. However, even if the facilitator is very skilled, group members can, at times, display disruptive behaviours. Table 16.1 illustrates some disruptive behaviours and a suggested facilitator response. Another way of minimising disruption is by splitting the group into small components (doing individual work, pairs or threes) so that they can focus on specific tasks without disruption.

Good facilitators make it look easy. The facilitator may or may not be a content expert. Many medical schools run groups with two facilitators whose knowledge complements one another's, for example a clinician and a scientist. It still requires as much preparation to facilitate a small group as giving a lecture – for the first time, plan roughly 4 hours' preparation for every 1-hour tutorial. The amount of work and skill required is often underestimated. Preparations include the environment, set, dialogue and closure, course reading material and prop preparation.

The facilitator sets the agenda and focuses the group on the issues. A good facilitator has the following qualities so the small group session runs smoothly:

- Competence and commitment
- Relaxed, interested and organised
- Maintains contact with learners – expert use of body language
- An active and expert listener
- A motivator
- Creates equal opportunities for all
- Pays attention to the self-esteem of all
- Has the ability to summarise what people say, rephrasing *incorrect* and emphasising *correct*
- Is non-judgemental
- Uses questions carefully
- Can give positive feedback.

Facilitating discussion

Alongside the group dynamics is the way the teacher feels the discussions should be managed. One way of thinking about what sort of small group session is appropriate is to consider whether it is closed (convergent) or open (divergent). It is important to understand the principal differences between these because the discussions and dynamics function very differently, therefore

inappropriate selection can lead to difficulties. Note that in longer sessions (e.g. half or one-day workshops) a mixture of approaches might be taken, depending on the purpose and task.

Closed discussion

In closed discussions, the facilitator maintains control throughout. All interactions take place through the facilitator. It can be compared to a well-run committee meeting where all discussion passes through the chairperson. This is achieved by careful attention to the layout of the room, classically in a horseshoe with each of the learners equally spaced (see Figure 16.1). The facilitator sits or stands in the middle so that he can see and interact with all the learners. This arrangement makes it quite difficult for conversations to spring up between the participants, and deliberately so. Closed questions by the facilitator, that is those with a right or wrong answer, help retain control.

The closed discussion is effective when the planned intention of the teaching session is:

- To impart new knowledge
- To revise what should already be known
- A definitive answer to posed questions
- A need to control time.
  Topics that might be included in a closed discussion are:
- How to manage a 'blue' patient
- The role of pulse oximetry
- The theoretical management of cardiac arrest
- The options available for postoperative pain relief.

Open discussion

The intention of an open discussion is that while the discussion may focus towards a specific question, the direction that the discussion will follow is unknown. Open discussions can be more challenging, as the technique encourages and even requires the participants to share their own opinions. However, open discussions are a powerful way of helping learners to work with a group, to put together coherent arguments and to learn to listen to others' points of view. It can be used as a way of demonstrating how others think and what acceptable behaviour is.

In order to facilitate this level of discussion, the format of the group is different. While the group leader focuses and guides the discussion, all members of the group need to have the opportunity to participate equally. They need to be at the same height, equally spaced in a circle. This allows everyone to see and speak to everyone else in the group. The facilitator forms part of the circle.

Managing this sort of discussion is much more difficult than in a closed group and time keeping can be a problem, especially with the use of open questions, which have no 'right' answer.

The open discussion works effectively when the planned intention of the teaching session is to help learners learn:

- To discuss a topic constructively
- To listen to others
- To function within a group
- From one other.
  Topics that might be included in an open discussion are:
- What constitutes informed consent?
- How cost influences treatment
- The value of 4-month rotations in postgraduate training
- Ethical issues.

Other ways of running small groups include buzz groups, brainstorming, fish bowl (where one group discusses in a circle and the other group observes) and snowballing (where small groups feedback to larger and larger groups). These methods all increase group interaction. See Figure 16.1 for different seating arrangements for discussion groups.

17 Clinical teaching: planning and design

Practice points

- The clinical setting is the most authentic for learning medicine but not always the most conducive to learning
- Teachers need to plan well and set out clear boundaries and expectations from learners
- Patient involvement is crucial but learning needs to be scaffolded and supported to protect all those involved

Box 17.1 Characteristics of a good clinical teacher

- Enthusiastic
- Interested in the wellbeing of students
- Capacity for dialogue as opposed to monologue
- Well prepared, organised and on time
- Teaching in the context of real patient cases
- Always developing ways to teach
- Behaves professionally

Figure 17.1 Clinical teaching environments (a) Family doctor consultation (b) Bedside teaching (c) Operating theatre

(a)

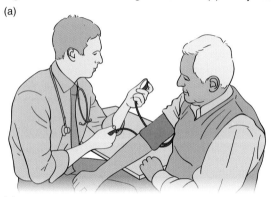

(b)

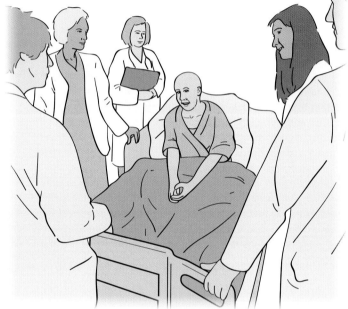

(c)

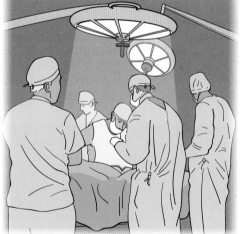

Figure 17.2 PACE model of graded assertiveness

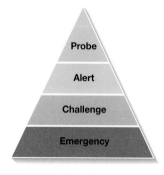

Probe

Alert

Challenge

Emergency

Figure 17.3 '# hello my name is' .... see http://hellomynameis.org.uk/

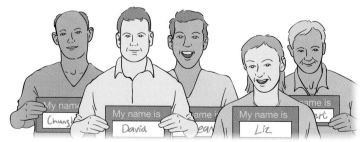

The clinical setting is the most authentic setting for students and doctors in training to learn and practise their clinical and communication skills. Doctors learn mainly from practice in a clinical environment and interactive techniques are most effective at changing physician behaviour. Therefore good teaching based in wards, clinics, surgery and by the 'bedside' is a vital aspect of learning clinical medicine (Figure 17.1). It integrates professionalism, communication skills, ethics and the development of practical wisdom (phronesis) with history taking and examination skills. Like all teaching, preparation is required. However, a key difference between clinical teaching and more formal classroom-based teaching is that the emphasis is on *facilitating learning* rather than *teaching*. Good clinical teachers have certain characteristics (Box 17.1).

Learning in clinical practice

Traditionally, exposure to clinical practice was in the later years of a medical school programme, but this is now changing with exposure to clinical teaching happening at many schools in the first year of the degree. When students are placed early on in clinical teams where they will be legitimate team members, not observers, learning is enhanced. Students can (and should) perform many roles, such as scribe or runner – valuable as initial learning experiences – before moving on to taking a history, doing an examination or learning to reason clinically. Such legitimate peripheral participation enables learners to engage with a community of practice and move along the novice to expert trajectory (Lave and Wenger, 1999). The primary unit of learning typically starts in the context of a clerkship or clinical team. Students within clerkships should have dedicated clinical support tutors and be fully prepared in terms of expectations and what is required of them to be self-directed learners as well as 'apprentices' and students. Enabling learners to work in the zone of proximal development (Vygotsky, 1978) requires learning to be scaffolded (structured) and learners to be challenged sufficiently so they can learn most effectively (see Chapter 5).

Creating a good learning environment

Learners (undergraduate and postgraduate) learn best when the environment is conducive to learning. At its simplest, this means their physical needs are met (e.g. space, rest, food and drink) as well as their emotional ones (e.g. a supportive relationship between the teacher, the wider team and learners). Clinical teaching can be the most intimidating for students, but patients themselves appreciate being involved in teaching. The teacher should prepare the session in advance with a lesson plan and the objectives of the session should be made clear to the learners (see Chapter 7).

Challenges and concerns

Challenges to clinical teaching include:
• A perceived conflict of interest for clinicians, as teaching is seen as separate from caring for patients
• Competing demands on clinicians' time such as roles in management and research
• Increasing numbers of students and a decreasing number of inpatients, therefore the opportunities for direct clinical teaching in hospitals are decreasing
• The clinical environment is not always conducive to teaching.
   Students also raise concerns about clinical teaching. These include (adapted from Spencer, 2010):
• Teaching often pitched at the wrong level with no clear objectives
• Passive observation rather than active participation
• Inadequate supervision
• Teaching by humiliation.

Set clear boundaries

Learners, especially those new to clinical practice, often struggle with understanding the culture and ways of doing things in different clinical environments. What may seem obvious to experienced clinicians (e.g. ward processes or hierarchy, theatre etiquette) can take some time for learners to understand. Whilst learners will have been taught about many aspects of clinical practice, it is not until you work somewhere that questions arise. Clinical practice brings together knowledge and understanding, practical skills and professional behaviours, and the hurly burly of service pressures can lead to learners sometimes doing things beyond their scope of practice or about which they feel uncomfortable. Anyone new to a clinical environment should always introduce themselves appropriately to all – patients and staff, and explain as clearly as possible who you are (Figure 17.3). It can be confusing for staff, learners and patients to work out who's who in the clinical environment. Many staff wear similar clothes (e.g. scrubs) and although someone may look like one thing (e.g. a child's parent) they maybe something else (a friend). Therefore never assume by appearances, always seek clarification.

Ethics in clinical teaching has been summarised as the **three Cs** (Spencer and McKimm, 2014): consent, choice and confidentiality. Clinical teachers are key role models for their learners; remembering the three Cs ensures that these are seen as fundamental pillars of good medical practice, not as options. Good practice is to inform patients that learners may be involved in their clinical care, and obtaining consent should be, 'a continuous process that begins with the first contact the service has with the patient' (Howe and Anderson, 2003 p. 327). Informing patients and seeking agreement should be done without the learner being present, then confirmed in the presence of learners (Howe and Anderson, 2003). Building in moment to moment opportunities for patients to say no to specific tasks that might be carried out by learners is another way of empowering patients and acknowledging their needs.

Spencer and McKimm (2014, p. 236) suggest that practical steps that help to maintain confidentiality include:
• Providing enough information to patients so they can assess and understand the boundaries of confidentiality
• Reassuring the patient and involving them in discussions
• Remembering that curtains around a bed or cubicle do not ensure silence
• Finding more private spaces to discuss intimate or distressing issues
• Discussing issues of confidentiality actively with learners as part of the preparation and debrief
• Obtaining permission for the use of images, sound recordings and extracts from case notes, particularly around anything that might identify a patient.

Sometimes learners may be asked to participate in what they may think is unprofessional practice, for example an intimate examination where they don't think the patient has given consent. This can create great pressures and dilemmas for learners. However, if a good learning environment is established from the outset, learners should be taught to challenge teachers on unprofessional and unsafe practices, for example using the PACE model in Figure 17.2 (see Chapter 28 for more on professionalism).

18 Clinical teaching: delivery

Practice points

- Teaching in clinical practice involves careful planning and consideration of the learning and clinical environment
- Learners need to be involved in clinical activities, either through allocation of increasingly complex tasks or purposeful observation
- A range of models are available for 'time poor' clinical teachers to facilitate learning opportunistically

Box 18.1 The one-minute preceptor model

- Get a commitment from the learner about the need to identify the nature of the problem: 'What do you think is going on with the patient?'
- Probe for underlying reasoning: 'What were the major findings that lead you to this diagnosis or decision? What else did you consider? What other information might you need?'
- Teach general rules (key teaching points)
- Provide positive feedback
- Correct errors in reasoning

Box 18.2 SNAPPS

S Summarise. Encourage the learner to present only the pertinent facts. Some of the background can be discussed with the analysis of the differential diagnoses

N Narrow differential diagnosis. The learner offers no more than 3 possible diagnoses

A Analyze the differential. Reviewing the pros and cons for each diagnosis allows the student to demonstrate analytic clinical skills

P Probe the preceptor. Here the student clarifies any difficult or confusing issues with the supervisor;

P Plan management. Developing a management plan requires an integrated clinical approach from the student

S Select an issue for self-directed learning. Reflecting on the case may reveal gaps in the learner's knowledge base. This final step requires the student to plan the steps to improve later performance

Figure 18.1 The Trialogue. Source: McKimm, 2008.

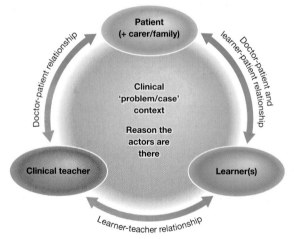

Figure 18.2 ISBAR

Medscape		
I	**IDENTITY OF PATIENT**	- Name/Age/MRN/ward/team
S	**SITUATION**	- Symptom/problem - Patient stability/level of concern
B	**BACKGROUND**	- History of presentation - Date of admission and diagnosis - Relevant past medical hx
A	**ASSESSMENT & ACTION**	- What is your diagnosis/ Impression of situation? - What have you done so far?
R	**RESPONSE & RATIONALE**	- What you want done - Treatment/Investigations underway or that need monitoring - Review: by whom, when and of what? - Plan depending on results/clinical course

Source: © 2011 The Fellowship of Postgraduate Medicine

Source: Thompson et al. (2011). Using the ISBAR handover tool in junior medical officer handover: a study in an Australian tertiary hospital. *Postgrad Med J* 87(1027), 340–344. Reproduced with permission of BMJ Publishing Ltd.

Medical Education at a Glance, First Edition. Edited by Judy McKimm, Kirsty Forrest and Jill Thistlethwaite © 2017 John Wiley & Sons, Ltd. Published 2017 by John Wiley & Sons, Ltd.

We touched on preparation in Chapter 17, both of environment and patients. Even with the best planning, however, this might have changed in a short time and so needs to be confirmed prior to any session.

Formal teaching sessions

Formal teaching sessions at the bedside, in outpatient and in theatre are addressed in other chapters; however, all have in common that at the start of the session the teacher should set the scene:

• **Ground rules** – the learners should be briefed on how the session will run (e.g. whether a full discussion will take place afterwards away from the patient) and professional behaviour (e.g. infection control).

• **Involvement and interaction** – questions and discussion should be encouraged throughout the session if appropriate.

• **Feedback** – learners should be made aware that feedback and/or reflection will take place throughout the session.

The Trialogue (Figure 18.1) provides a structured way for teachers to manage both the learner–teacher and the doctor–patient relationship (McKimm, 2008). The clinical teacher simultaneously attends to the triadic dialogue by:

1 Facilitating conversations between learner and patient (so that the learner can learn from the patient whilst developing their own relationship with the patient)

2 Maintaining their own relationship with the patient through carrying out clinical activities and conversations

3 Enabling the learner to learn by explaining, illustrating and demonstrating what is going on.

Purposeful observation

It is not always appropriate for learners to carry out examinations or procedures themselves and much can be gained from observing more senior or expert practitioners. However, observation needs to be purposeful so that learners (particularly those new to a clinical environment or procedure) can gain the most out of watching someone else do something. Rather than saying 'just watch me', it is useful to ask the learner to observe specific aspects of care and ask for their comment afterwards, for example asking them to observe what specific (closed) questions you asked a patient as opposed to general (open) questions, and what information was elicited from each type.

Teaching on the run

When time is limited, you may need to be more opportunistic in seeking out 'teachable moments'. This is often known as 'teaching on the run' (e.g. Lake and Ryan, 2004). Opportunistic learning episodes occur frequently within clinical settings, but these are not always used to their full potential. Opportunistic teaching is often misinterpreted by both learners and teachers as not requiring preparation or forethought but, as with all teaching, this not true. The following questions should be asked (and can be quickly thought through):

• How long will the learners be with you?
• What have they done before?
• What will the learners do next?
• What do the learners expect to happen?
• What are the intended learning outcomes of this placement?
• How will the learners be assessed?
• Who else is involved in teaching and learning at this point?
• What are your expectations of them?
• Where can teaching take place?
• Who else might be involved in teaching?
• What special resources can you offer?

The range of teaching techniques and methods that can be employed in each setting is varied. Often learners don't realise, if the teaching is not formal, that teaching is happening. Therefore:

• Be explicit about learning, explain how it will occur and when it is taking place.

• Ask/reflect on what learners have learned at the end of each episode.

Teaching in chunks

Lake and Ryan describe two models of 'quick teaching'. The One-Minute Preceptor Model (OMP) is a way of incorporating teaching into a patient-focussed clinical encounter (Box 18.1). This approach was developed in the US in 1992 as the Five-Step Microskills Model of clinical teaching. The OMP model focuses the teaching encounter on the learner's reasoning, while simultaneously gathering the necessary components of the history and physical examination. This is similar to asking open-ended questions of patients to gather the history, rather than jumping right into direct questioning. This model allows the preceptor/teacher to assess the learner's knowledge and reasoning, and provide key messages for learning. Other methods of teaching in quick digestible chunks include asking questions, reviewing patients that the student has seen and then discussing your diagnosis and management plan The SNAPPS model (developed for outpatient clinics) is set out in Box 18.2. These teaching methods provide a way of teaching when the focus is on patient care. Small chunks of teaching can be very effective, particularly when they are set in an overall context in which learners are expected to participate in learning.

Ward round teaching

Wards rounds are often seen as a place to get work done and learners as a distraction to the real job of patient care. However, with a little forethought, ward rounds can be used effectively as excellent learning opportunities without detriment to the care of patients and not taking too much time. Plans for future ward rounds that can help educate as well as 'get the work done' of caring for patients include:

• Assigning each learner roles for the day – scribe, prescriber, examiner and history taker, which can be rotated over the week.

• Dividing the team in two, with each taking opposite ends of the ward and meeting in the middle to discuss all patients.

• Teaching on only two or three patients for that day, explaining this to the learners and the patients.

• Having an 'investigation of the day' (e.g. ECGs, X-rays or blood results) that teaching will concentrate on.

• Peer teaching – asking a more senior trainee or student to go through something with a more junior colleague, e.g. national asthma guidelines and meet at the next patient with asthma.

• Using handovers or handoffs as an educational tool, teaching communication strategies (e.g. **ISBAR**, Figure 18.2) and role modelling professional behaviours.

19 Simulation: planning and design

Practice points

- Simulation enables learners to practise clinical and communication skills in a safe environments before working with *real* patients
- It also has benefits for health systems in that complex or crisis situations can be experienced and practised
- A wide range of simulation activities, equipment and contexts exists – choice of simulation is directly related to learning needs, not the technology available

Box 19.1 The range of simulated experiences

- Games, classroom scenarios
- Wet labs using human or animal tissue
- Simulated patients: actors, healthy volunteers, standardised patients
- Computer-generated virtual reality simulators (two dimensional and three dimensional)
- Manikins and models of varying complexity: from part task trainers, such as cannulation arms, to 'complete' bodies such as Simman™
- Mock facilities including a simulated operating theatre, emergency departments, delivery suite, ambulance and wards

Box 19.2 Rationale, pedagogical and safety advantages of using simulation-based training

The simulation setting:

- Provides a safe environment
  - for learners without risk of harming the patient
  - that is fully attentive to learners' needs
  - for training individuals and multiprofessional teams
- Can be adjusted according to learners' needs
- Enables exposure to
  - gradually more complex clinical challenges
  - rare emergency situations where time is an important factor
- Provides an opportunity for
  - experiential learning
  - repetitive training, deliberate practice
  - individualised, tailored learning
  - formative assessment, debriefing and feedback
  - stimulating reflection
  - learning how to learn
  - summative assessment

Source: Østergaard and Rosenberg, 2013. Reproduced with permission of John Wiley and Sons.

Box 19.3 Best practice features of simulation

- Formative feedback (feedback for learning) during simulation
- An opportunity for deliberate (purposeful) and repetitive practice
- Curriculum integration
- Outcome measurement
- Simulation fidelity (i.e. it must be as lifelike as possible)
- Skills acquisition and maintenance
- Mastery learning
- Transfer to practice
- Team training
- High-stakes testing
- Instructor training
- Educational and professional context
- A variety of conditions and range of difficulties

Source: McGaghie *et al.*, 2010; Issenberg *et al.*, 2005.

Figure 19.1 Simulation

Figure 19.2 Simulation activities integrated into the learning programme. Abbrev: WPBAs, workplace-based assessments.

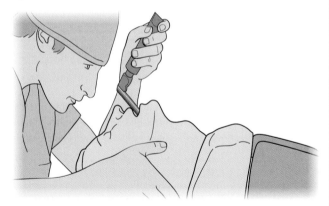

| Knowledge e-learning | Basic skills on part task trainers | Complex skills virtual reality Simulated scenarios | Supervised clinical practice Log books/WPBAs |

Most learners and practitioners will be trained and assessed using some form of simulation, and the use of simulation is now seen as routine in health professions' education. Advances in technology have led to very lifelike simulators for patients, surgery procedures and full-scale mock-ups of wards, theatres, delivery suites, ambulances and emergency departments. Many include software so that the simulator's reactions depend on learners' actions. There are many advantages to simulator training. The most obvious is that learners can practise as often as they like and whenever they want (within reason) without harming a patient.

How is simulation used?

Simulation training extends from part task trainers, or procedural training, to the experience of full clinical situations (e.g. cardiac arrest). Box 19.1 lists the range of simulated experiences.

Simulated parts of the body can be used, for example, for cannulation, feeding, catheterisation or rectal examination. Some skills are practiced in a wet lab where animal and human tissue can be used, for example, for suturing. Basic (low-fidelity) manikins are used for teaching basic and advanced life support (Figure 19.1). High-fidelity manikin simulators with a vast number of programmed interactions and physiological responses can be used for individual or team scenario training. Scenario simulation provides an excellent opportunity for interprofessional education with the ability to train real teams from work environments. High-fidelity simulators also include those that are used for laparoscopy, endoscopy or where virtual reality is employed. Some of these sophisticated simulators have forced feedback (haptic) systems, which enable the learner to 'feel' the endoscope going around the splenic flexure or to manipulate the 'baby' in a complicated delivery.

Benefits of simulation teaching

The use of simulation in health professions' education has been shown to have benefits for learners, for development of clinical practice and practical (technical) skills, for patients and for health systems (Riley et al., 2003). As well as facilitating the acquisition of routine skills, simulation also allows safe (for the learner and the patient) exposure to rare diseases/conditions, critical incidents, near misses and crisis situations (Box 19.2). Reflecting the experience of the airline, nuclear and other high-risk industries, evidence is accumulating that patient safety standards and non-technical skills (communication, leadership, teamworking etc.) improve following simulator training (McGaghie et al., 2010).

Simulation and learning

Simulation works most effectively when it is designed to meet curricular outcomes, includes realistic and relevant content, interesting and engaging learning methods and prepares learners for working in the clinical context in terms of activities, skills and competencies (Issenberg et al., 2005). Box 19.3 lists the best practice features of simulation as identified in two systematic literature reviews.

Simulation helps skills acquisition, maintenance and assessment in the move from novice to expert (Dreyfus and Dreyfus, 1985). The key element here is building simulation activities into learners' progression (Figure 19.2). For example, students must practice and master female catheterisation skills and pass an assessment before going on clinical rotations, or doctors in training might have to provide evidence of competence in resuscitation using a simulator before interacting with patients. Learners can therefore have their first encounter with patients at a higher level of technical and clinical proficiency, which protects patients.

Special types of simulation

Many people imagine simulation as being carried out in purpose-built skills labs or high-fidelity simulation suites, but many activities use simulation routinely to achieve learning outcomes without such costs. Examples include the use of actors in teaching communication skills, role play, standardised or expert patients assisting with practical skills examinations, and the use of peers to learn anatomical landmarks or practise examination skills.

Distributed simulation

Some of the biggest constraints to widespread simulation training are cost, expertise and access. One group has tried to address these issues by identifying the key aspects of the different clinical environments (e.g. the operating theatre or intensive care unit) that are needed for learning and then replicating these in a portable environment that can be set up in a short space of time and a small area. This is 'distributed simulation' (DS) (Kneebone et al., 2010), where inflatable, portable simulations can be erected in places of work and immersive simulations can be run. In addition to providing more easily accessible training, this kind of technology is much cheaper.

Tang et al. (2013) describe the key components of DS as:
• A self-contained, immersive environment which can be closed off from its surroundings
• Providing the minimum necessary cues to recreate a realistic clinical context (e.g. equipment, people, sounds – conversation, monitor sounds,)
• Simple, user-friendly recording and playback equipment, often using mobile devices
• Practical, lightweight, portable components, which can be put up quickly by a small team
• Flexibility to recreate various settings according to requirements.

Peripatetic simulation

The increasing emphasis on the ability to bring the simulation to the learner, rather than learners having to travel to a centre, has also been replicated by other initiatives. These include 'man in a van' (Simvan), where the equipment is mobile and simulation is taken to the learner and ambulances, which are set up as real ambulances, but are learning facilities which go to different locations. However, such developments need trained faculty to travel with the equipment, which can limit its use.

20 Simulation: delivery

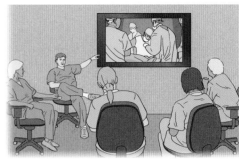

Practice points

- Effective simulation is designed around a believable scenario
- Teachers have responsibility for ensuring and maintaining a safe environment where mistakes can be made and lessons learned
- Simulation education comprises deliberate practice, feedback and the structured debrief

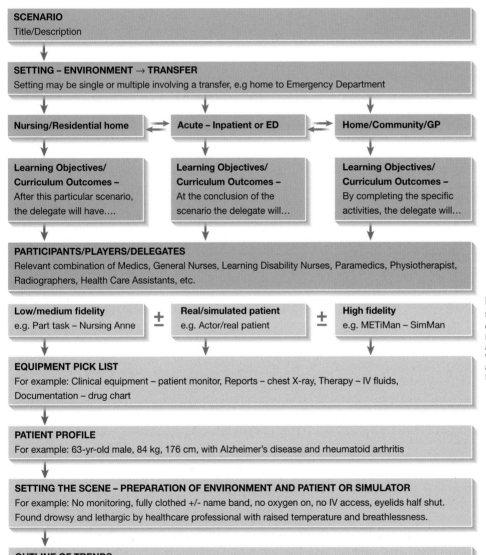

Figure 20.1 Key to successful simulation is the scenario that is designed and delivered. Source: Forrest K, McKimm J, Edgar S (eds) (2013) *Essential Simulation in Clinical Education*. Wiley Blackwell. © Copyright NHS Yorkshire and the Humber Clinical Skills Team 2012. Reproduced with permission.

SCENARIO
Title/Description

SETTING – ENVIRONMENT → TRANSFER
Setting may be single or multiple involving a transfer, e.g home to Emergency Department

Nursing/Residential home ⇌ **Acute – Inpatient or ED** ⇌ **Home/Community/GP**

Learning Objectives/ Curriculum Outcomes – After this particular scenario, the delegate will have….

Learning Objectives/ Curriculum Outcomes – At the conclusion of the scenario the delegate will…

Learning Objectives/ Curriculum Outcomes – By completing the specific activities, the delegate will…

PARTICIPANTS/PLAYERS/DELEGATES
Relevant combination of Medics, General Nurses, Learning Disability Nurses, Paramedics, Physiotherapist, Radiographers, Health Care Assistants, etc.

Low/medium fidelity e.g. Part task – Nursing Anne ± **Real/simulated patient** e.g. Actor/real patient ± **High fidelity** e.g. METiMan – SimMan

EQUIPMENT PICK LIST
For example: Clinical equipment – patient monitor, Reports – chest X-ray, Therapy – IV fluids, Documentation – drug chart

PATIENT PROFILE
For example: 63-yr-old male, 84 kg, 176 cm, with Alzheimer's disease and rheumatoid arthritis

SETTING THE SCENE – PREPARATION OF ENVIRONMENT AND PATIENT OR SIMULATOR
For example: No monitoring, fully clothed +/- name band, no oxygen on, no IV access, eyelids half shut. Found drowsy and lethargic by healthcare professional with raised temperature and breathlessness.

OUTLINE OF TRENDS
Combination of (1) (2) (3) or all (1) Communication > scripts/direction
(2) physiological > low-, medium- or high-fidelity programming (3) psychomotor skills

DEBRIEFING OVERVIEW
To include – Review of learning objectives against performance, key indicators of achievement against objectives and discussion around tagged events that occur during simulation

As with all learning activities, it is vital to plan the learning carefully with clear aims and learning outcomes. However, because of the specific requirements of simulation, additional activities need to be undertaken if it is to work well.

Delivering simulation activities

Key to successful simulation is the scenario that is designed and delivered (see Figure 20.1). Depending on the needs, level and number of learners (and available facilities and faculty), a suitable scenario needs to be devised. This should be tested or piloted to make sure that the timing, learning outcomes and participants' and others' roles work in practice.

A simple scenario might be that learners have to assume that a whole body manikin is an elderly patient requiring sitting up in bed, making comfortable and then taking admission information. Another might be a simulated patient (actor) to whom the learner has to break bad news. More complex scenarios might vary in the complexity of the patient's (or family's) needs/condition; a scenario with two or more parts where the condition deteriorates, new information is provided or might involve more people taking different roles, to very complex scenarios involving whole teams, and/or high-fidelity simulators and confederates (actors) who might play the part of patients, family members, other professionals and health service managers.

The course/session

Both participants and faculty need to be familiar with the setting and equipment being used before embarking on the scenario. This may involve a prebriefing or training and sending out materials or information prior to the event. Eppich *et al.* (2013) suggest the following needs to be planned in advance and attended to throughout the course or session:
• Foster informal discussion and conversations
• Introductions and icebreakers
• Use first names (both faculty and participants) for the duration of the session to break down hierarchy
• Learn people's names (labels may be useful)
• Give overview of the session/course
• Provide clear ground rules about process and expectations
• Foster psychological safety
• Orientate to the simulation environment and equipment (location of equipment, manikin, roles of participants, rules of engagement)
• Carry out briefing to the scenario, clarify everyone's roles (including observers), assumptions, clinical knowledge
• Carry out simulation
• Feedback and debrief
• Prepare any follow up activities/materials.

Much of the philosophy of simulation education is based on deliberate practice with appropriate feedback and reflection (both during and after the event).

Deliberate practice

Deliberate practice refers to time spent on a specific activity designed to improve performance in a particular aspect of practice and is more effective than simple unstructured practice. There is a consistent association between the amount and the quality of deliberate practice and performance in domains as varied as chess, music and sport (Ericsson, 2004). Deliberate practice means that there is effort involved as well as some form of feedback, whether through self-assessment, from the simulator or observation by another person.

Feedback

The absence of learner feedback is the greatest single factor for ineffective simulation training. In this context, feedback refers to the specific information provided to the learner about their performance against a defined standard or competency to help improve future performance. For example: 'You put exactly the right pressure on the chest when you were doing the compressions; however, the timing was not consistent and you need to practise again to get the right rhythm going'. See Chapter 37 for more information on feedback.

The structured debrief

One of the key elements of the simulation experience is the debrief. Debriefing enables the transformation of the simulation experience into learning (which hopefully can then be applied in practice) through reflection, feedback and discussion. The debrief provides an opportunity for a facilitated reflection through conversation to explore issues, and help the learner identify gaps or the need for more learning in their knowledge, skills or professional behaviours. Whereas feedback should not explore motives or rationale for actions (or omissions), debriefing does. It can therefore be very challenging to the learner as it is more critical and needs to be carefully facilitated within a safe learning environment.

Eppich *et al.* (2013) suggest the structured debrief comprises the following components:
• Preparing the physical space – debriefer and participants usually sit in a circle
• Setting the stage and clarifying expectations
• Allow for initial emotional reactions (e.g. venting, defusing) to help participants come out of role by asking an open question such as 'how do you think that went?'
• Describe the main events and primary issues to be explored so everyone is on the same page
• Discuss participants' performance: what was done well, what could have been improved
• Application of learning to future practice
• Summary of learning points.

One model used in debriefing is Debriefing with Good Judgement, developed by educators at the University of Cambridge, MA, which uses the principles of advocacy-inquiry (Rudolph *et al.*, 2006). In this model, the facilitator gives feedback on performance and also shares their point of view or judgement and inquires about the learners' perspective. This gives the opportunity for a professional conversation to occur, which goes much deeper than simple feedback and promotes the learners' reflection and insight by surfacing the learners' reasons for their actions. For example:

I noticed that you kept looking at your colleague when you were doing the chest compressions and not at the monitor, did you notice this yourself? And why do you think you did this?

Such an observation might reveal that the learner was lacking in confidence in the technique, was seeking approval from the colleague or was expecting the colleague to count compressions for them. Whatever the reason for the actions, this opens up opportunity for a conversation that helps the learner perform better next time.

A very useful aspect of higher-fidelity simulation is the ability to play back videos of the scenario that has been played out to an individual or team. With the widespread use of wireless and mobile technologies, this is an increasingly flexible tool which can be carried out in situ or remotely. Unlike verbal feedback from an observer, being able to play back a video provides tangible, detailed and specific evidence of what the learner did or did not do or say. In addition insight into how they behave under stress (getting angry, withdrawal, making mistakes) can be a valuable and powerful learning tool.

21 Patient involvement in education

Box 21.1 Nomenclature

Patient-educators may be referred to as:
- Clinical teaching or patient teaching associates
- Gynaecological teaching associates (GTAs) are women who teach students intimate examinations (e.g. pelvic, breast).

Box 21.2 Spectrum of involvement

Six educational roles:
1. Cases based on patients' stories available for case-based learning on paper or electronic; includes virtual patients
2. Simulated or standardised patients
3. Patients share their stories and experiences with learners as part of an educator-defined curriculum and learning outcomes
4. Patients as educators involved in teaching and assessing learners
5. Patients as educators and equal partners in planning and development
6. Patients involved at an institutional level, including student selection

Adapted from Towle *et al.*, 2010.

Figure 21.1 Level of patient involvement. Source: Adapted from Tew *et al.*, 2004.

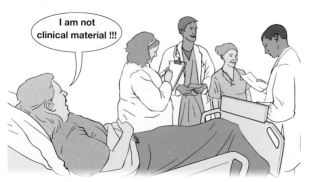

Passive patient level 1

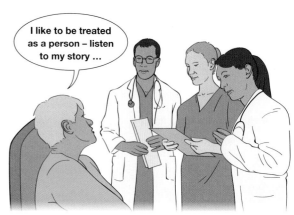

Active patient level 2 and 3

Medical Education at a Glance, First Edition. Edited by Judy McKimm, Kirsty Forrest and Jill Thistlethwaite © 2017 John Wiley & Sons, Ltd. Published 2017 by John Wiley & Sons, Ltd.

The patient voice in education

For many decades, patients have been thought of as the passive objects of medical education. Indeed Abraham Flexner, whose report on medical education in North America led to widespread change in curricula in the twentieth century, referred to patients as 'clinical material' (Flexner, 1910). Such language is no longer acceptable in this era of patient partnership and patient-centred health care. While patients and service users are involved in diverse ways in many health and social care professional programmes, the patient voice is still relatively silent in medical curricula and teaching (Health Foundation, 2011).

There is evidence that patient involvement enhances knowledge, skills, attitudes and behaviours of learners, clinicians, educators and patients themselves; however, there are few data relating to longer-term outcomes on health and practice (Health Foundation, 2011).

The rationale for patients having a greater involvement in education is that it is patients, their families and their community who are experiencing the health and social problems and conditions that influence their decisions to consult professionals. Patients are experts on their own perspectives, and living with illness or long-term conditions. They contribute rich stories of accessing health care, interactions with health professionals and organisations, and how their social environment impacts on their well-being: all of which may be outside a health professional or medical student's own experience. Thirty years ago Tuckett and colleagues described patient–doctor interactions as meetings between experts and advocated that sharing ideas on both sides was important during consultations (Tuckett et al., 1985).

Note that this chapter refers to the patient as this is the nomenclature associated with the medical profession and thus medical education (see Box 21.1). However when patients are involved in learning, educators should ask them how they would like to be addressed and the terminology to use. Clinicians and educators also need to be wary about suggesting that everyone is a patient at some time. While this is true, health professionals experience health care in a different way to lay people for many reasons including power differentials. The **patient voice** needs to be heard from all levels of society, particularly from those sectors whose voices are frequently ignored.

Levels of patient involvement

Patient involvement ranges from none at all to full partnership (see Figure 21.1). It is important to acknowledge the role of all patients with whom learners interact during clinical placements. These patients are in the healthcare system predominantly for diagnosis and management. Students learn from and about patients with facilitation from clinical teachers and appropriate health professionals. However, in these situations patients may have no active role in deciding what students should be learning, nor in guiding such learning into areas that the patients wish to discuss. There are also simulated patients (such as actors), who work to help learners with communication and clinical skills, again usually under the guidance of educators and health professionals.

Increasing the level of patient involvement means that patients have a greater voice throughout a programme. This is in line with greater patient engagement within a health service and acknowledgement of patients' opinions in terms of governance; for example, there are now lay people involved in the UK's General Medical Council's (GMC) professional activities. With greater patient involvement, students and doctors in training learn with and from patients.

The Cambridge framework

This framework (Spencer et al., 2000) was devised to help educators categorise the level of patient involvement. There are four questions (adapted from Spencer et al., 2000):

Who: who are the patients, where do they come from, what is their culture and what are their stories, who else is involved such as family, carers and social networks?

How: how are the patients to be involved, what will be their role (active or passive), how long will they be involved, and what supervision may be required?

What: what are the learning outcomes, the learning activities, and assessment?

Where: where will the interaction and learning take place, for example in a community setting (including patients' homes), in hospital, in a clinic?

To the above we can also add: what sort of training, if any, do the patients require; will patients receive funding such as honoraria/expenses; is such funding sustainable; and how will the involvement be evaluated?

Preparing to involve patients

It is instructive for medical educators to consider the current level of patient involvement in their programmes (Figure 21.1 and Box 21.2). Where do patients fit on the ladder or spectrum of involvement in your institution? If you want to enhance the patient voice, you need to define the reasons for doing this. This is an important step for all concerned, including patients, who ideally should be included in planning from the beginning. Ethical issues should be considered in relation to consent and confidentiality: for example learners should not discuss details about patients working as facilitators, educators or mentors on social media or other contexts.

There may already be links between your wider institution and community groups. Some schools in the university may have community liaison workers, or similar, who can be important sources of information for the medical school. While patients may be recruited as individuals through adverts in hospital and primary care centres, it is more productive for larger-scale involvement if educators work with robust, stable community organisations that have the capacity for sustained partnerships (Towle and Godolphin, 2015). Patients and community groups should benefit from the interactions as much as the medical school or postgraduate organisation and learners.

All parties working and learning in new ways will need orientation. Specific training will be needed for those patient educators who will be giving feedback to learners on specific skills such as communication, and those who will be assessing in Objective Structured Clinical Examinations (OSCEs) and similar clinical examinations.

22 Ward-based and bedside teaching

Box 22.1 Learning can be facilitated through different techniques

- Thinking aloud
- Demonstrating – for example an examination technique
- Generating questions about the evidence base (and asking one student to research the answer and then present later)
- Having students review a patient first, think about the problem(s), and then present their management plan (including presenting to and interacting with the patient)
- Discussing similarities and differences between patients to encourage pattern recognition and clinical reasoning
- Giving feedback and encouraging students to give feedback
- Asking patients for feedback
- Telling clinical stories to illustrate an evidence-based point
- Encouraging **noticing**
- Asking what three things people learned at the end of a ward round (reflection)
- Recommending specific further reading

Box 22.2 Ward-based learning examples

- Dedicated bedside teaching
- Ward rounds – business and teaching
- Grand rounds and board rounds (formal discussion of patients and cases away from the bedside)
- Shadowing – senior students are attached to the intern/foundation doctor whose job they will have once qualified
- Student assistantships – designed to help transition from student to doctor (final year students work alongside interns/foundation doctors; this is longer than shadowing and learning depends on location, supervisor and opportunities)

Source: Burford *et al.*, 2015.

Figure 22.1 Orientation

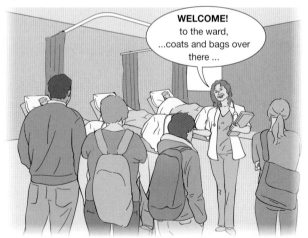

Figure 22.2 Thinking aloud

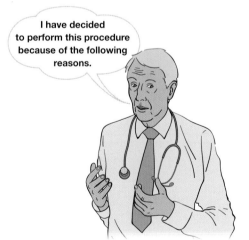

The provision of frequent opportunities for students to visit, observe and carry out appropriate tasks on hospital wards is important. The majority of new graduates (interns/foundation year 1) will work in hospitals and be the first-line medical professionals. Along with medical students, they therefore need to be acculturated to the ward environment in order to feel comfortable interacting with sick patients and working with other health professionals. More senior doctors in training may have longer rotations, but will still need orientating to each new ward or department. Note that you should build in for a competence dip at all times of transition, no matter how senior a practitioner (e.g. Wilkinson and Harris, 2002).

While students should be encouraged and timetabled to spend time on wards across a variety of specialties (for example acute medical, surgical, paediatric, elderly medicine and day wards), medical educators need to combine student-directed learning with both formal and opportunistic bedside teaching. As with all learning and teaching, good preparation and orientation is required.

Orientation

Learners should be orientated to their hospital and to specific wards (Figure 22.1). Students should have an understanding of hospital personnel, what uniforms people wear, where the student space is for coats, studying etc., which bathroom facilities they may use and where they may buy drinks and food (and eat and drink).

While many students may have had experience of being on wards as visitors, workers (for example as healthcare assistants), volunteers and even patients, as learners without a specific role they may feel lost and possibly in the way, as surplus to patient care requirements. Clinical teachers should prepare students for the ward environment. Students should be reminded how to dress (and to wear the appropriate identification), what equipment they should carry and what is available for their use on the ward, how they may recognise the person in charge (usually a nurse) and introduce themselves, and how patients they may approach are identified.

Medical schools vary in how students are attached to wards and medical teams, to whom they report and who is responsible for monitoring attendance and performance. Learners may feel awkward and reluctant to ask for help and feedback unless they are welcomed by teaching staff, who are not necessarily always medical doctors. It is important to advise students that timetabled formal teaching sessions may have to be postponed if clinicians have unexpected priorities elsewhere. As they progress through their education and training, learners should be given increasing responsibilities.

Clinical teacher preparation

Ward-based teachers are a diverse population. Some may be nurses or other health professionals specifically employed to facilitate students in their learning of clinical skills – helping them transfer from a skills lab or simulation to a real-life setting. Others are doctors undergoing further training, who may have an interest but frequently little formal training in education. Specialists usually have a responsibility within a teaching hospital to include students on their team. Career medical educators may also debrief learners following clinical placements. Medical educators are frequently involved in the professional development and mentoring of clinical educators.

Bedside teaching focuses on patients, who usually appreciate being involved in helping learners develop their skills. Before a formal teaching encounter, the teacher or facilitator should identify appropriate and willing patients that fit with the learning outcomes for the session. Teachers need to know what those learning outcomes are and the point in the medical programme the learners have reached. Some teachers will meet the same group of learners over time but this is not always the case. They should also explore what the learners themselves hope or expect to learn.

At the bedside

How many learners with their facilitator fit comfortably around a bed without intimidating patients? This should be small group teaching with two to perhaps six learners.
• Consent to participate in teaching should be obtained from the patient.
• The learners should be briefed on how the session will run (e.g. whether they will be asked to elicit histories, carry out an examination, where the discussion or debrief will take place, whether a full discussion will take place afterwards (away from the patient) and reminded about professional behaviour (e.g. infection control, respect, confidentiality).
• Introductions are important – including the patients.
• Involvement and interaction – questions and discussion should be encouraged throughout the session; again this should include the patient.
• Feedback – learners should be made aware that feedback and/or reflection will take place throughout the session.
• Patients should be advised that they too can ask questions and that some discussion may not relate directly to them.
• Facilitators need to be aware of patient comfort and when a session needs to be ended if patients are tiring.

Learning and teaching tips

Many learners will have portable electronic devices, which they may be encouraged to use to look up guidelines, drug dosages and interactions, and evidence. Some of these techniques may not necessarily be considered 'teaching' (e.g. thinking aloud [Figure 22.2], or telling a clinical story over coffee), which is why an explicit emphasis should be placed on learning, rather than teaching, in a busy ward environment (see Box 22.1). Other techniques may be used to teach in chunks when time is limited including the One-Minute Preceptor Model (Neher et al., 1992) (see Chapter 18).

Being observed can be an intimidating experience, but is vital for receiving useful feedback and learning. It is important to involve all the learners during a session so that some do not feel picked on. There is no place in contemporary medical education for teaching by humiliation.

Lack of space on wards can be a problem. Teaching and debriefing is not always appropriate at the bedside but there may not be a suitable location for this to take place. Corridor education is not ideal as corridors are public spaces and sensitive information may be overheard. Board rounds, around the whiteboard with patients' details on, may be an alternative (see Box 22.2), or holding a case-based discussion away from the ward (see Chapter 31).

23 Learning and teaching in ambulatory settings

Practice points

- Ambulatory settings are those other than by the bedside (i.e. clinics, family medicine surgeries)
- Students need to be actively involved in tasks rather than simply observing
- Longer placements in community settings facilitate students feeling part of the team

Box 23.1 Broad learning outcomes in ambulatory settings

- Understanding patients' and carers' experiences
- The patient journey
- Patient-centred approaches
- Communication skills
- Clinical reasoning
- Focussed interviewing
- Evidence-guided investigations
- Patient management
- Shared decision making
- Informatics
- Continuity of care
- Health promotion and disease prevention
- The primary healthcare team
- Understanding of health professionals' roles and responsibilities

Figure 23.1 Models of consulting

Computer Table **P** **Dr** **St**
Student as an observer

Computer Table **P** **St** **Dr**
Student being observed

Computer Table **P** **St** **St**
Student being observed by a peer

Computer Table **P** **St** **St** **Dr**
Student being observed by doctor and peer

Computer Table **P** **St**
Parallel consulting

Computer Table **P** **Dr**

P = Patient
Dr = Doctor
St = Student

In this chapter we concentrate on locations where patients are ambulatory, that is they are not in-patients or bed bound but attending a clinic or surgery in either the community, out-patient department (OPD), radiology or day procedural suites. While medical students frequently interact with patients on wards without direct supervision in order to clerk and elicit histories, in ambulatory settings students should have specific tasks provided. In community settings such as general practice, patients may be invited to the surgery specifically to interact with students; at other times students' learning activities focus on patients attending for consultations and care. It is important when developing ambulatory learning and teaching opportunities that learners are actively involved in some way, not just passive observers, sitting in the corner of the consulting room. As doctors in training become more skilled and experienced, teaching techniques will shift from direct supervision or observation of consultations, to their seeing more patients alone, for example in parallel consulting (Figure 23.1).

Medical Education at a Glance, First Edition. Edited by Judy McKimm, Kirsty Forrest and Jill Thistlethwaite © 2017 John Wiley & Sons, Ltd. Published 2017 by John Wiley & Sons, Ltd.

Early patient contact

Ambulatory settings are ideal for early patient contact within a medical programme. Until about two decades ago, medical students rarely interacted with patients in the preclinical years. In 1993 in the UK, the General Medical Council stipulated that more of the medical curriculum should be moved into the community (community-based medical education) (GMC, 1993) and this was partially achieved by students spending time in general practices from their first year. Students may also interact with patients and families in their homes and community settings. Such meetings and reflection typically form part of family projects or personal and professional development (PPD) modules (Box 23.1).

In general practice, and sometimes in the OPD, junior students elicit patients' stories rather than the more formal medical histories learned in later years. Learning outcomes relate to students gaining a greater understanding of patient experiences of health and illness, the patient journey and how conditions may change over time. Students also practise their communication skills, particularly the patient-centred approach, which involves their exploring people's ideas, concerns, expectations and values (Stewart *et al.*, 1995; Thistlethwaite and Morris, 2006). Usually students interview patients without being observed; they may do this in pairs or larger groups, and sometimes the groups may involve students from other health professions (**interprofessional learning**). They then debrief with a tutor, either back at the medical school (perhaps their PPD facilitator) or with a GP from the practice to which they are attached.

Students may also learn clinical skills in clinics, where they attend with a tutor and examine patients under supervision, usually focussing on a specific body system in each session. Patients may be invited to attend because they have a particular condition or physical sign.

All involved in these activities need to be fully briefed and orientated to the learning. Patients need to be recruited and consent to participate in teaching. If they are travelling they should receive expenses. Some schools may also pay patients for their time and expertise. As this may be the first time students are involved with *real* patients, they need to be aware of the dress code and etiquette required, as well as discuss the concept of confidentiality. Tutors and GPs (who may receive payment) should be aware of the learning outcomes, what the students have already covered and the assessment of the activity.

Models of learning and teaching

In the *clinical years*, students are attached to ambulatory settings for longer periods of time. This may be the relevant OPD for a hospital-based specialty during a specific rotation (e.g. surgery, gynaecology, paediatrics). Students also undergo attachments in primary care/general practice for varying lengths of time, depending on the medical school. Increasingly, doctors in training spend time in community and ambulatory settings; however, this varies with specialty and country.

Patterns of general practice rotations

- One day per week for one semester, or 1 year, or 2 years etc. Students may be attached to more than one practice during this time, e.g. urban and semirural.
- Several consecutive weeks: often between 4 and 8 within 1 year and at the same practice. Frequently includes half to 1 day per week at the medical school for central teaching with all GP-based students.
- Longitudinal placements involve students spending up to 1 to 2 years in the same general practice with planned rotations into secondary care.

When planning ambulatory education, the first few days should involve orientation to the clinic, the personnel and the patient care delivery system. Learners should spend a few sessions sitting in on appropriate consultations. Patients need to consent to the presence of students and practices must have processes in place to do this. However, so this observation is not a totally passive process, the health professional conducting the consultation should agree relevant tasks with the student. GPs and others need to block off protected time during the session for discussion and de-briefing.

Questions and tasks during observation periods

- Notice how patients are greeted and how they respond.
- What seems to help patients present their stories?
- How long are patients allowed to speak before the health professional asks another question?
- How does the computer affect the consultation? Is it used in a patient-centred manner?
- Look for emotional cues and how the health professional responds.
- In what ways are consultations ended?

Active participation

Students are always eager to do things; they soon become de-motivated if only observing. If there is a spare room a student should be asked to see patients prior to their appointment with the doctor or other professional. This could be in pairs or alone. The consultation may be video-taped for later discussion if the technology is available. The patient needs to consent (and this will of course add time to their attendance). The student should be given a specified time and then report back on what has been elicited to the professional. Ideally, the report is given in the presence of the patient so facts may be clarified. The professional then takes over the consultation in discussion with the student as appropriate, involving the patient in the usual way. The student may be supervised performing the appropriate physical examination and senior students may be able to discuss management plans. Patients may be asked to give feedback to the student if they feel comfortable to do this and there is time.

A second model is that the student is observed during the whole interaction. Feedback is a dialogue between the health professional and the student, involving the patient as appropriate.

Obviously, these models take time and, in general practice, may result in having to cut some appointments from a session. This has ramifications for the practice and patients, so agreement of the whole practice is necessary when deciding on whether to host students. Clinical teachers within ambulatory settings also require professional development for education. This also adds to their time commitment.

24 Teaching in the operating theatre

Practice points

- The operating room is a good context for learners to work interprofessionally, learn technical skills and follow the patient journey
- Observation, thinking aloud and role modelling are all useful learning models in the operating theatre
- Operating rooms are good for teaching one-to-one (TONTO) which has both benefits and disadvantages

Figure 24.1 Example form to give to a student to observe the 'teacher' in theatre

		Comments on behaviour observed
Task management	Prioritising	
	Identifying and utilising resources	
Teamwork	Co-ordinating activities with team members	
	Exchanging information	
	Assertiveness	
	Assessing others' capabilities	
	Supporting others	
Situation awareness	Gathering information	
	Recognising and understanding	
	Anticipating	
Decision making	Identifying options	
	Balancing risks and selecting options	
	Re-evaluating options	

Figure 24.2 Role modelling

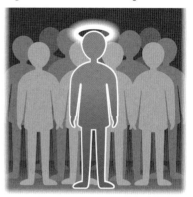

Figure 24.3 Attributes of a negative role model

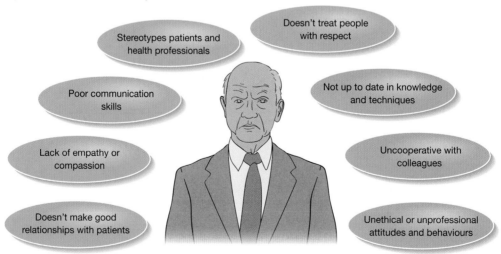

Stereotypes patients and health professionals

Doesn't treat people with respect

Poor communication skills

Not up to date in knowledge and techniques

Lack of empathy or compassion

Uncooperative with colleagues

Doesn't make good relationships with patients

Unethical or unprofessional attitudes and behaviours

Operating theatres or the operating room (OR) can be a scary place for learners. More than other places in a hospital or community practice, it can feel alien and uninviting. Like other teaching encounters, introductions and orientation should be completed before learners enter theatres, including where to get changed into theatre attire, where to leave bags and simple procedures signed off/completed before being in the workplace such as hand washing and scrub training.

Benefits of operating room teaching

In-theatre training can be with surgeons, anaesthetists and other healthcare professionals. Although limited technical skills can be taught and learned in the earlier years of education and training, for more junior learners the reasons for being present have to be made explicit both to the learners and teachers. The reasons for learning can include:

1 Understanding how and why patients go to theatre. A learning objective might be to observe the contexts in which patients are cared for immediately prior to surgery and to understand the procedures undertaken. Anaesthetists are particularly well placed to teach about topics such as identifying the sick patient, fluid management and pain control.

2 Participating as much as is possible and allowed (with consent) in procedures occurring in theatre, such as suturing and cannulation.

3 Facilitating an understanding of cases from a surgical and anaesthetic perspective. Doctors in training will often prepare patients for theatre and they need to understand what is needed and why, for example specific blood tests and investigations for procedure.

4 Working and learning in multiprofessional teams. Here the learning outcomes relate to inter- and multiprofessional team working, development of personal and professional attitudes and values and understanding the role and responsibilities of members of professional groups.

Specific learning models

Some specific models for learning, while applicable to other areas, are especially useful in the OR setting.

Observation

More so than other workplaces, students have to observe in theatres for a lot of their time there. Often this is perceived as a waste of time by students and sometimes staff as well. However, demonstrations are what many clinicians do all the time in their clinical practice. But without making it clear to the student that this is a learning opportunity, the learning can be missed. This can be as simple as stating something like, 'I would like you to watch how I take a history/ examine the patient/perform this procedure. Concentrate on what questions I ask/what I look for/how I interact with theatre colleagues. Afterwards I would like you to summarise what you observed and then we will discuss it further.' Figure 24.1 illustrates a form that can be given to senior students to observe non-technical skills.

The expert 'thinking aloud'

As experts, some of our clinical judgements can appear to be so intuitive as to be unteachable. As a teacher you may be asked how you just *knew* something. This is a bit like trying to explain how you drive a car, broken down into its constituent parts, and can be difficult. Sound clinical reasoning and judgement at critical points in time is a valuable skill for students to learn. How did you know that the patient was sick? The answer of 'gut feeling' is not helpful and is not supported by the literature on expert practice. Gut feelings ('rapid intuition') usually involve the immediate recognition of a constellation of signs (visual, auditory etc.) that fit into the pattern that matches with your previous experience. Often, as a clinical teacher, the simple act of thinking aloud can help learners understand the steps you are taking when coming to a decision and management plan, and this facilitates learning.

Role modelling

Role modelling is teaching by example (Figure 24.2). Poor role modelling (Figure 24.3) can have a powerful impact on the informal and hidden curricula, which are described in Chapter 6. There are three categories of role modelling in medicine:
- Clinical competence
- Teaching skills
- Personal qualities and professionalism (e.g. compassion, integrity, enthusiasm, quest for excellence).

Role modelling is a good way to demonstrate professional behaviours and can be used to teach other aspects of patient care, for example infection prevention and communication skills. Many doctors in difficulty may be perpetuating behaviours they have observed go unchallenged in senior colleagues.

Teaching one-to-one

Teaching one-to-one (TONTO) can be a luxury for a busy clinician (Gordon, 2003). However, operating theatres and general practice, by virtue of space constraints, are settings where TONTO is often a necessity. There are many advantages of TONTO for both the learner and the teacher:
- No competing demands of other learners and the teacher can pitch material at the appropriate level
- Provides the opportunity to explore the learner's understanding of material at a deeper level than in a group setting.
- Feedback can be more timely and specific.

Disadvantages include:
- There can be blurring of roles for the clinician between teacher, mentor, counsellor and friend.
- Student and teacher personality differences can be a complicating factor.
- There may be a lack of social learning support from fellow learners.

The effective application of TONTO demands particular attention to the nature of the relationship between the teacher and learner, something Lyon described as sizing up (Lyon, 2004). This mutual process can lead to feelings of trust and legitimacy, which in turn validates the learner's presence as a legitimate peripheral participant in the community of practice (Lave and Wenger, 1999).

Not all learners are equally confident in new environments and the professional hierarchies encountered in specialised settings can make teaching didactic rather than inclusive. By thinking about the processes that are familiar to the healthcare professionals within the operating theatre it becomes possible for the teacher to encourage learner participation and interaction.

25 Interprofessional education

Practice points

- Interprofessional education (IPE) helps future and existing health professionals work better together to improve patient care
- IPE can be offered at different levels: exposure, immersion and mastery
- IPE improves collaborative practice, which allows health workers to engage any individual whose skills can improve health goals

Figure 25.1 The four-dimensional framework for IPE. Source: Lee, *et al.*, 2013. Reproduced with permission of Australia and New Zealand Association of Health Professional Educators.

Dimension 1: identifying future healthcare practice needs

This dimension seeks to connect health professionals' practice needs to new and changing workplace demands in all health sectors. Curriculum considerations take into account global health and educational reforms; how these link to the development of knowledges, competencies, capabilites and practices; as well as local institutional delivery conditions.

Dimension 2: defining and understanding capabilities

This dimension describes the knowledges, capabilities and attributes health professionals require. This component addresses how changing health services impact on expertise, identities and practice, which ultimately impacts upon the training and preparation of future health professionals.

Dimension 4: supporting institutional delivery

This dimension focuses on the impact of local university structure and culture on the shaping of curriculum design and delivery, such as timetabling, logistics and entry requirements.

Dimension 3: teaching, learning and assessment

This dimension pertains to the development of appropriate learning, teaching and assessment experiences, all of which have been guided by the messages inherrent within D1 and D2.

D1 Future orientation of health practices — Graduates — **D4** Institutional delivery

Practitioners — Multidimensional curriculum reform — Educators

D2 Knowledges, competencies, capabilities, practices — Learners — Teaching, learning and assessment approaches and practices **D3**

Figure 25.2 Interprofessional education model. Source: Charles *et al.*, 2010. Reproduced with permission of Taylor & Francis.

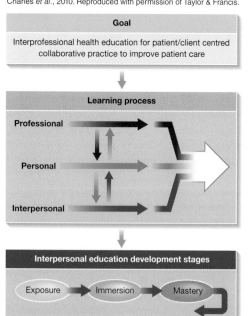

Goal

Interprofessional health education for patient/client centred collaborative practice to improve patient care

Learning process

Professional

Personal

Interpersonal

Interpersonal education development stages

Exposure → Immersion → Mastery

Box 25.1 Tomorrow's doctors

Learn effectively within a multiprofessional team:

- Understand and respect the roles and expertise of health and social care professionals in the context of working and learning as a multiprofessional team.
- Understand the contribution that effective interdisciplinary team working makes to the delivery of safe and high-quality care.
- Work with colleagues in ways that best serve the interests of patients, passing on information and handing over care, demonstrating flexibility, adaptability and a problem solving approach.
- Demonstrate ability to build team capacity and positive working relationships and undertake various team roles including leadership and the ability to accept leadership by others.

Note: multidisciplinary, interdisciplinary and multiprofessional are sometimes used synonymously.

Source: General Medical Council, 2009.

Medical Education at a Glance, First Edition. Edited by Judy McKimm, Kirsty Forrest and Jill Thistlethwaite © 2017 John Wiley & Sons, Ltd. Published 2017 by John Wiley & Sons, Ltd.

The most frequently used definition for IPE is: 'occasions when two or more professions learn from, with and about each other to improve collaboration and the quality of care' (CAIPE, 2002). The prepositions 'from, with and about' imply that the education is interactive and equitable.

Rationale

As health and social care is delivered by a diversity of professionals, some of whom work in well-defined teams and some in looser collaborations, 'medical' education should no longer be restricted to medical students. No single health professional can have the knowledge and skills to provide care for every patient, family or community. In particular, the rising incidence of chronic and long-term conditions, such as cardiovascular disease, diabetes, dementia, and mental health problems, requires that clinicians understand one other's roles and responsibilities, and can work together to provide optimal care. Logically, learning together enhances working together; the rationale behind the interprofessional education (IPE) movement.

The World Health Organization's (WHO) *Framework for Action on Interprofessional Education and Collaborative Practice* (2010) is a good summary of the reasoning behind both IPE and interprofessional practice. Educators should also refer to the Lancet Commission's call for changes to medical education (Frenk *et al.,* 2010) to influence curriculum committees. This international group of 20 professional and academic leaders developed a shared vision and strategy for the education of health professionals, highlighting the need for team-based care, and advocating for IPE as part of a continuum of training. In addition, the WHO's guidelines for health professionals' education recommend that institutions should consider implementing IPE but with the proviso that IPE requires more research into its outcomes: 'IPE may be resource-efficient in a way that allows more health workers to be educated; there is a need to obtain much better evidence in institutions with both programmes and resources available to support the necessary research' (WHO, 2013, p. 44).

> Collaborative practice happens when multiple health workers from different professional backgrounds work together with patients, families, carers and communities to deliver the highest quality of care. It allows health workers to engage any individual whose skills can help achieve local health goals.
> Canadian Interprofessional Health Collaborative, www.cihc.ca

The interprofessional curriculum

The four-dimensional framework (Figure 25.1) is a useful tool for curriculum development (Lee *et al.,* 2013). IPE is logistically difficult and there needs to be added educational value in organising large numbers of students from different schools and often different universities to learn together. Therefore the **learning outcomes** must be such that they can only be achieved through interaction and through the interprofessional mix.

> ## Commonly included competencies / domains
> * Team work
> * Communication
> * Roles and responsibilities
> * The patient
> * Learning/ reflection
> * Ethical/ attitudes
> Source: Thistlethwaite and Moran, 2010.

Learning activities

The University of British Columbia (Vancouver) model of IPE (see Charles *et al.,* 2010) is a useful way to think about developing learning activities. It has three levels (Figure 25.2):

1 Exposure: early stages of learning such as group work, discussion of roles, use of videos as prompts, case studies, online modules, healthcare team challenge etc.

2 Immersion: simulation and clinically based activities, small groups of students interviewing patients, training wards, rural integrated placements etc.

3 Mastery: postqualification, incorporating interprofessional working into one's professional practice (Figure 25.2).

While IPE is not solely about teamwork, students do need to be given suitable opportunities to learn about teams and working with other professions. Interprofessional clinical placements are examples of work-integrated learning (WIL) designed to aid the integration of theory and practice (Orrell, 2006). Students therefore require a prior theoretical platform on which to build their clinical learning and orientation to the people working within clinical environments (Thistlethwaite, 2015b). Because of the nature of clinical education, students will have diverse experiences with varying exposure to and immersion in teamwork experiences. Observation of healthcare teams in action is not sufficient; students need to become members of teams and have experience of the complex tasks and boundary challenges of decision making and service delivery (Orrell, 2006). Situated and experiential learning is enhanced through continuity of location and supervision (Thistlethwaite *et al.,* 2013).

Assessment

To emphasise the importance of interprofessional education and collaborative practice (IPECP) to students, assessment of learning outcomes is necessary. As IPE is ideally an interactive, collaborative learning process, team-based formative assessment is best practice, with observation and feedback to enhance further learning. Portfolios (also called interprofessional passports) are useful tools for students to provide evidence of achieving outcomes, but there may be issues relating to reliability and feasibility if used for summative purposes. Multisource feedback (MSF) forms can be included, which require students to obtain feedback on their teamwork from peers and the different health professionals with whom they interact. Some institutions are trialling team OSCEs (T-OSCE) or interprofessional OSCEs (iOSCE) with relevant simulation activities (Simmons *et al.,* 2011; Symonds *et al.,* 2003).

Interprofessional facilitation

The delivery of successful IPE requires expert facilitators who have interprofessional experience beyond previous uniprofessional working. IP facilitators should have most of the following attributes:

* Understanding of the relevance of and evidence for IPE
* Expertise in team work theory and team building
* Experience of working in a healthcare team
* Awareness of boundary issues in health care
* An understanding of the process of professional socialisation
* Skills in negotiation and conflict resolution.

Evaluation and research

Medical and health professional educators require a deeper understanding of the outcomes and processes of IPE. Evaluation is an important part of curriculum planning and more in-depth research studies are needed to explore how and why IPE may inform healthcare delivery and patient outcomes.

26 Reflective practice

Practice points

- Reflection is a key element of professional development and practice
- A number of models exist to structure reflective conversations and writing
- Evidence of reflection is increasingly required for students and practising doctors
- Structured opportunities for purposeful reflection need to be built into programmes from the start

Box 26.1 Definitions

- Common sense reflection: day-to-day thinking after a situation that has affected a person (Moon, 2004); 'we reflect for a purpose' (Moon, 1999, p. 4).
- 'Active, persistent and careful consideration of any belief or supposed form of knowledge in the light of the grounds that support it and the further conclusion to which it tends' (Dewey, 1933, p. 9).
- 'A purposeful, questioning approach…requires us to challenge preconceived notions or ways of working… and our taken for granted assumptions' (Crawley, 2005, p. 183).

Box 26.2 Types of reflection

Cognitive based reflection

- What the learner knows
- Defining learning needs
- Intrinsically motivated learning
- Deep approach to learning
- Stimulation of prior learning
- Accommodation and assimilation

Reflection for personal development

- Developing professional identity
- Membership of communities of practice
- Dealing with significant events, achievements, suffering, death, errors, job stress

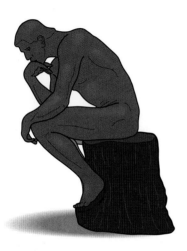

Figure 26.1   Framework for reflection. Source: Gibbs, 1988.

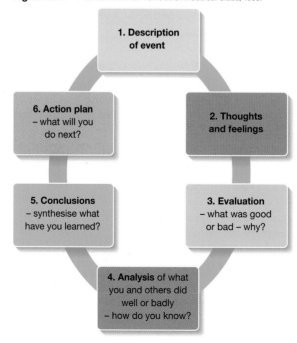

Medical Education at a Glance, First Edition. Edited by Judy McKimm, Kirsty Forrest and Jill Thistlethwaite © 2017 John Wiley & Sons, Ltd. Published 2017 by John Wiley & Sons, Ltd.

Reflection has been an important activity in higher education for many decades. However, it was in the 1970s and 1980s when the idea of reflective practice became more widespread through work on experiential learning (for example Kolb and Fry, 1975) and the influential book *The Reflective Practitioner* (Schön, 1983). In medical education, the aim of reflection is to help learners (and indeed teachers and clinicians) improve their practice and learn from experiences, both adverse and positive events. The literature has expanded to include how to teach and learn reflection and, more controversially, how to assess reflection. Reflective portfolios, which have been used in nursing for some time, have been introduced for both formative and summative assessment by many medical schools. Yet there are still a number of definitions of reflection and the concept remains relatively ill-defined (Box 26.1).

Reflection is a rich, individually focused process and in almost every case will include elements of cognitive-based and personal development-based activity (Box 26.2). Teachers, facilitators and course developers need to think about the purpose of reflective activity when they introduce it to their learners to ensure that optimum support is given and optimum outcomes achieved. Whatever the learning outcomes desired from reflective activity, learners will be more likely to achieve these if support from a suitably trained tutor or mentor is offered. In time, and with training, learners can act as mentors to one other.

Reflection and professional behaviour

Being a professional rather than a technician implies reflection (see Chapter 28). Schön (1983) and Greenwood (1998) have stressed different types of reflection that educators may refer to when encouraging learners to reflect in and on practice:

- **Reflection before action:** planning what you are going to do before an activity or situation (prospective)
- **Reflection in action:** thinking about what is happening 'right now – in the moment' and how you are reacting; enables you to change what you are doing or your responses if necessary
- **Reflection on action:** thinking after the event or activity (retrospective) and how you might change in a similar situation in the future
- **Reflection for action:** purposeful reflection to help define new goals or learning needs (prospective).

Boud *et al.* (1989) stress the *affective* component of reflection and the strong emotions it may trigger, which involves three components:

- Returning to an experience (recalling significant events)
- Attending to or connecting with the feeling associated with the experience
- Evaluating the experience in the light of existing knowledge or new understanding.

Learners need to be aware of their feelings, and facilitators should be alert to these. Encouraging learners to talk about their emotions in a safe and supportive environment is important.

The experiential learning cycle

Following the work of Dewey (1933) and Kolb (1984), experiential learning theory looks at learners' acquisition of knowledge and skills and their awareness of what they do and don't know (metacognition). The **experiential learning cycle** has been published in many forms and can be another useful aid to reflection to introduce to learners (see Chapter 5). It starts from the premise that learning begins with a concrete experience, and learners then are encouraged to reflect on the situation analytically. During this process they might think about what happened and how well their current knowledge enabled them to understand what was going on. Learners should be encouraged to reflect on what they have learned from the experience and what gaps in their learning have emerged in order to plan future learning. Learning in response to knowledge gaps that have been self-identified is intrinsically motivated and is likely to be carried out with a deep approach (Grant, 2013) so that learners make meaning from learning rather than acquiring isolated facts. In the last stage of the cycle, learners experiment with applying their newly acquired knowledge and/or skills to situations similar to the initial experience.

The experiential learning cycle is a model of how learning may occur, rather than an account of what happens to each individual learner. In many cases, the various stages of the cycle may not take place in the smooth cyclical way that the model suggests. For example it may only be when learners' thoughts are stimulated by another experience that they are able to achieve the realisation that makes it possible for them to carry out abstract conceptualisation that, in turn, enables them to gain new insights.

Reflection for personal development

When students are first introduced to reflective learning they may feel uncertain what they have to do (Grant, 2013). Reflective templates offer a structure, which can make early attempts at reflection easier and can 'walk' students through the reflective learning cycle (e.g. Figure 26.1). Learners should experience the benefits of reflective learning early, and the learning tasks should not be too onerous. It is important to nurture learners' spontaneity. If a learner using a reflective template based on experiential learning comes across a challenge to their beliefs and values, then they should be encouraged to write about and reflect on this.

Students (or anyone) embarking on their first reflective learning encounter need reassurance. They may fear that it is their thoughts and values that are being examined, rather than their learning. In order to support their sense of self-efficacy, they should receive the help and support they need to see themselves as competent reflective learners. Computer-based templates can provide a small amount of just-in-time information for each point in the reflective cycle.

Facilitating reflection

Small group work may be structured around a significant event or case-based discussion as part of regular meetings with supervisors, mentors or peers. These professional conversations are aided by defining outcomes, a clear structure, prompting questions and a set time frame to help set clear boundaries around the conversation (McKimm, 2009).

27 Teaching clinical reasoning

Practice points

- Clinical reasoning explains how doctors think and make decisions
- It is important to acknowledge that diagnostic tests are subject to error and humans have cognitive biases
- Evidence-based medicine is the art of applying best available evidence *to an individual patient* – 'evidence' is often applied incorrectly by novices
- Simple frameworks can be used for making clinical decisions

Box 27.1 Teaching probabilities*

Modelling: 'making connections' or 'putting two and two together' with gathered information using clinical knowledge

A 40-year-old male was admitted to hospital with vague abdominal pains and a fever. He drank alcohol to excess. His white cell count was slightly raised and he had proteinuria 1+. A diagnosis of urinary tract infection was made and he was started on antibiotics. What kind of reasoning might follow the presentation of this case?

- Urinary tract infections are uncommon in 40-year-old men
- One of the commonest causes of proteinuria 1+ is fever and this is not diagnostic of a urinary tract infection
- Gastritis and pancreatitis are more common causes of vague abdominal pains in males who drink alcohol to excess
- Pancreatitis commonly causes fever
- A serum amylase should be requested. (This patient did have acute pancreatitis.)

*Understanding diagnostic tests: a Bayesian approach uses all the relevant information from the history and physical examination (pretest probability), and incorporates information about the sensitivity and specificity of the test to estimate post-test probability.

Figure 27.1 Clinical knowledge

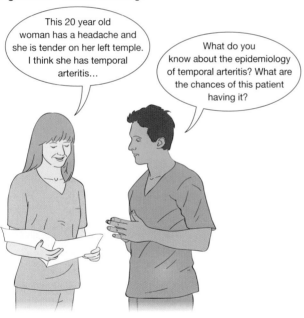

Figure 27.2 Cognitive biases

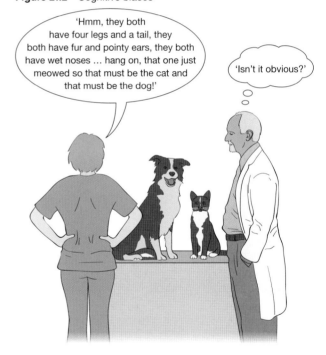

Figure 27.3 Decision-making strategies

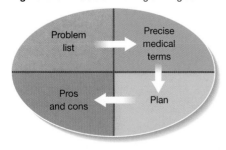

Even with twenty-first century medical technology, history and examination remain the cornerstone of diagnosis. However, the failure rate in diagnosis is estimated to be 10–15%, highest among specialties that deal with undifferentiated presentations (Trowbridge and Graber, 2015). The most common reason for mistakes in diagnosis is errors in clinical reasoning. Dr Pat Croskerry, Professor of Emergency Medicine and expert in clinical reasoning, points out that, 'Usually, it's not a lack of knowledge that leads to failure, but problems with the clinician's thinking. Common illnesses are commonly misdiagnosed. For example, physicians know the pathophysiology of pulmonary embolus in excruciating detail, yet because its signs and symptoms are notoriously variable and overlap with those of numerous other diseases, this important diagnosis is missed in a staggering 55% of fatal cases.' (Croskerry, 2013, p. 2445). It is therefore vital that all learners understand and can demonstrate effective clinical reasoning – or *how doctors think*. This chapter briefly summarises five key components of a clinical reasoning curriculum or course.

Clinical knowledge

It is vital that students are taught clinical knowledge and skills in the context of diagnosis (Figure 27.1). For example, most students can recite risk factors for cardiovascular disease. They should also be able to use this knowledge to estimate a patient's clinical probability of having coronary artery disease when he/she presents with chest pain. They should have a basic understanding of Bayes Theorem from clinical vignettes taught alongside 'dry' epidemiological and physiological facts (Box 27.1). Likewise for examination, students are taught the typical signs of deep vein thrombosis (DVT). However, they should also know that examining a leg for a possible DVT can be as accurate as tossing a coin. Learners require a foundation of clinical knowledge in order to be able to reason effectively.

Understanding diagnostic tests

There is no such thing as a perfect test. All tests are subject to sensitivity and specificity, operating characteristics and factors other than diseases that can influence test results (for example, age or ethnicity). The probability that a patient has a disease depends on the pretest (clinical) probability and the sensitivity and specificity of the test (Sox *et al.*, 2013). Students need to understand that fractures and strokes can occur with normal radiological investigations, or that significant emphysema can be present with normal spirometry, for example. A study of common as well as illustrative investigations can be used to teach key points.

There is no such thing as a perfect test:
- Sensitivity is the ability of a test to detect true positives.
- Specificity is the ability of a test to detect true negatives.
- Tests that are very sensitive detect most diseases, but also generate lots of false positives.
- Tests that are very specific establish the diagnosis when the result is positive, but may miss significant pathology.
- All tests have a sensitivity and a specificity: *tests do not make a diagnosis – clinicians do.*

Psychology and cognitive biases

Cognitive psychologists have described the human mind's vulnerability to cognitive biases, false assumptions and a range of other reasoning failures. There are two principal ways in which our brains manage and process information, widely known as System 1 and System 2. System 1 is intuitive, fast and automatic – the **rapid cognition** used commonly by experts, but in many situations is highly vulnerable to error. System 2 is analytical, slower and effortful (Kahneman, 2012) (Figure 27.2). Psychologists suggest we spend 95% of the time in System 1 mode. Clinicians are often unaware of the limitations of human performance that affect their clinical reasoning and decision making. Thinking and decision making can be affected by context and other factors such as:
- Personality type and decision-making style
- Overconfidence
- Night work
- Overwork, stress, interruptions
- Cognitive load (too many decisions to make)
- Peer pressure/group think
- Strict hierarchy in teams

Understanding how we think, factors that can affect thinking and being mindful of one's own thinking are vital aspects of effective clinical reasoning. Being aware of the different cognitive biases that exist and when they are most likely to occur, coupled with purposeful practice and feedback from an expert, can help students learn effective clinical reasoning skills (Cooper *et al.*, 2016).

Evidence-based medicine

Evidence-based medicine is the application of best available evidence to an individual patient, taking in to account not only their physiological characteristics but also their preferences and concerns. Doctors need to know how to access evidence, how to critically appraise it, and how to apply and communicate it to real patients. They also should learn a healthy scepticism for sponsored information. An awareness of how standardisation can improve quality and safety should be covered, and they should be aware of important organisations that produce national guidelines for common clinical conditions.

Decision-making strategies

Students can be taught a simple framework for reasoning through a case and coming up with a management plan. One example is the Four Ps (Figure 27.3):
- **Problem list:** the ability to identify key clinical data from history, physical examination and (sometimes) initial test results is a key step in clinical reasoning. Some problems require a differential diagnosis, but not necessarily, and most patients have more than one problem.
- **Precise medical terms** (e.g. pleuritic chest pain): these help 'chunk' information, which aids memory storage and retrieval, so it is important to frame the problem list using precise medical terms.
- **Plan:** make a plan for each problem.
- **Pros and cons:** then filter the plan through its advantages and disadvantages, for example a treatment could be contraindicated due to another problem, be more likely to cause harm than benefit, or be contrary to the patient's wishes.

Sound clinical reasoning is required for safe clinical care, so teachers should teach reasoning skills as well as knowledge and skills.

28 Professionalism

Box 28.1 Roles of a doctor

The **UK General Medical Council** defines three main roles for doctors:

1. The doctor as a scholar and a scientist
2. The doctor as a practitioner
3. The doctor as a **professional**

The **Australian Medical Council** has four domains:

1. Science and scholarship
2. Clinical practice – doctor as practitioner
3. Health and society – doctor as a health advocate
4. **Professionalism** and leadership

The **CanMEDs framework** lists six roles of the medical expert:

1. **Professional**
2. Communicator
3. Collaborator
4. Manager
5. Advocate
6. Scholar

But what/who is a professional?

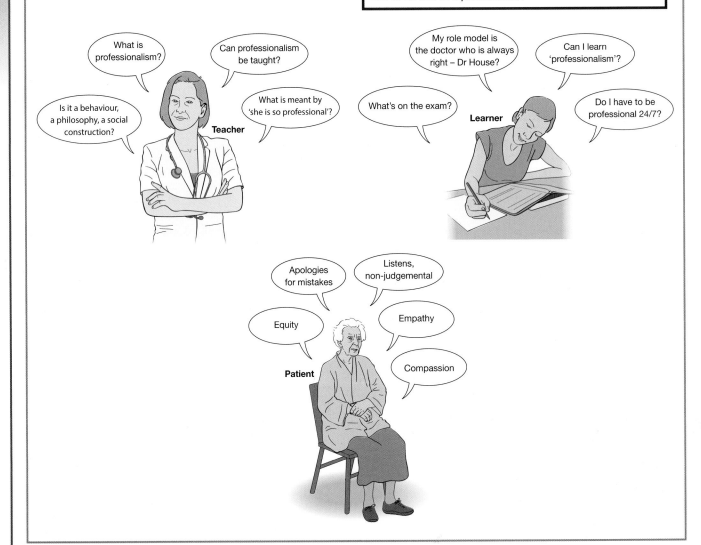

Professionalism is now a required component of medical school curricula in many countries, as stipulated by accreditation bodies such as the General Medical Council (GMC) in the UK (Box 28.1). The GMC (2009) states that 'The principles of professional practice set out in Good Medical Practice must form the basis of medical education' and a set of learning outcomes based on these principles has been defined. While professionalism may be conceptualised in different ways, there are many similarities across medical schools in the way it is learned and taught.

Definitions

> **Professionalism**: 'the competence or skill expected of a professional' (Oxford English Dictionary, 2016).
> A **professional** is:
>
> A member of a profession – from the Latin *profiteri,* to avow or profess; for example many doctors *profess* the Hippocratic oath when they qualify.
> 'A reflective practitioner who acts ethically' (Hilton and Slotnick, 2005).

In medical education literature the following longer definition of profession is useful for discussion with medical students: 'an occupation whose core element is work based upon the mastery of a complex body of knowledge and skills. It is a vocation in which knowledge of some department of science or learning or the practice of an art founded upon it is used in the service of others. Its members are governed by codes of ethics and profess a commitment to competence, integrity and morality, altruism and the promotion of the common good within their domain' (Cruess *et al.,* 2004, p. 76). Professionalism involves a 'social contract' between the profession and society, allowing professionals a degree of autonomy and self-regulation while, in return, society expects that professionals are accountable to those they serve, their profession and society (Cruess *et al.,* 2004).

The code of conduct or ethics – in other words how to behave – is the essence of professionalism. Medical education introduces students to the code of their chosen profession, including ethical and legal requirements. Professionalism is taught through formal and informal activities, and students are expected to learn the correct way to behave. Moreover, professionalism and professional behaviour is now assessed through a variety of means (see Chapter 42).

Professionalism courses

Whether professionalism can be taught has been debated in the education literature. Certainly, learning outcomes can be defined for certain aspects of professionalism, and these form the basis of what is commonly called personal and professional development (PPD) in the curriculum. However, professionalism should not be thought of as a separate course: professional behaviours should be encouraged, discussed and integrated throughout a programme.

Key aims of professional development during medical school are:

- To enable students to understand the origins of professionalism and the proper set of responsibilities of the medical profession.
- To instil and nurture in students the development of personal qualities, values, attitudes and behaviours that are fundamental to the practice of medicine and health care.
- To ensure that students understand the importance and relevance of these concepts, demonstrate these qualities at a basic level in their work and are willing to continue to develop their professional identity.

The most common components of formal professionalism courses include:
- Ethics and the duties of a health professional
- The law applied to health professional practice
- The role of the regulatory body (e.g. the General Medical Council in the UK; the Australian Health Professional Regulatory Authority (AHPRA) and the medical boards in Australia)
- Communication (not only with patients but also with colleagues/other health professionals; and not only oral but written and online)
- Teamwork and collaboration, leadership
- Self-care
- Cultural awareness and cultural competence
- Reflective practice
- The use (and abuse) of social media
- Patient safety and whistle blowing.

Small group work may also include discussion about professional attributes such as altruism, empathy and compassion. Some schools include teaching on professional autonomy, error and patient safety, evidence-based practice and values-based practice under professionalism.

Learning and teaching methods and principles

Formal learning activities should provide context and be relevant to clinical practice, linking theory and practice. In the first year, facilitators may use media portrayals of doctors and other health professionals as examples for discussion. Cases should ideally be grounded in the real world of patient and professional interaction, the local health services, and the experiences that students and doctors encounter in daily practice. Clinicians and patients should be involved in both the planning and delivery of the teaching – they can bring their own examples of practice-based encounters and dilemmas. Learning and teaching should also be based as much as possible on the experiences and concerns of learners, particularly when they begin clinical practice. Everyone who interacts with learners is a role model and needs to demonstrate exemplary professional behaviour. Common professionalism dilemmas for clinical students include: what to do after observing poor patient care; being abused as a student; and lack of consent (see Rees *et al., 2013* for teaching and learning relating to professionalism dilemmas).

29 Peer learning and teaching

Box 29.1 Planning for peer learning and teaching

- Who are the learners?
- Who are the teachers?
- How are the teachers to be recruited?
- Define required attributes and competencies for teachers
- Provide rationale to all involved
- Size of groups
- Identify appropriate curriculum learning outcomes
- Identify appropriate learning activities
- Plan timetabling
- Plan education development for teachers
- Build in observation and feedback
- Decide on appropriate assessment for learners
- Plan and implement evaluation

Box 29.2 Checklist items of the WATCH: the Warwick Assessment insTrument for Clinical TeacHing for peer observation

- Promotes active engagement of learners*
- Communicates effectively with learners
- Maintains polite and considerate attitude with learners
- Expresses enthusiasm towards teaching and learning
- Teaches concepts and skills in an organised manner
- Demonstrates clinical competence appropriate for the stage of training
- Adjusts teaching to learners' needs
- Demonstrates appropriate use of teaching aids and resources
- Provides constructive feedback to learners
- Stimulates reflection and problem-solving skills
- Is able to teach in diverse settings and involves patients in teaching (if relevant)
- Demonstrates professional and ethical conduct
- Avoids favouritism, criticism and discrimination
- Remains up-to-date with knowledge of developments in the field
- Is a good role model

* 'learners' substituted for 'trainees' in the original.

Source: Haider *et al.*, 2015. Reproduced with permission of Taylor & Francis.

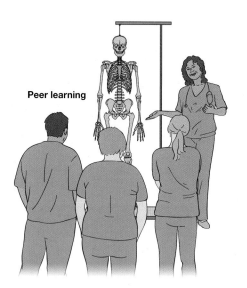

Peer learning

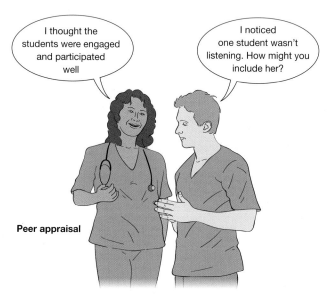

I thought the students were engaged and participated well

I noticed one student wasn't listening. How might you include her?

Peer appraisal

Medical Education at a Glance, First Edition. Edited by Judy McKimm, Kirsty Forrest and Jill Thistlethwaite © 2017 John Wiley & Sons, Ltd. Published 2017 by John Wiley & Sons, Ltd.

Medical education is a life-long process for clinicians. Doctors must (and do) continue to learn throughout their careers, from their first day as a medical student to the moment they retire. They learn from many sources: senior clinicians and health professionals; role models; journals and websites; their students, patients and peers. Learning from peers is often informal and serendipitous. It also occurs during small group and problem-based learning sessions, although the facilitator is not usually a peer in these situations or, if they are, has had training in facilitation.

Formal **peer** and **near-peer** teaching is now becoming more common. A peer acts as a tutor, assisting colleagues who are the tutees (Ross and Cameron, 2007). Peer or near-peer teaching occurs when learners and teachers are at similar stages of training but typically separated by one or more years (e.g. junior and senior medical students). Cross-level training occurs when learners and teachers are at adjacent stages (e.g. medical students and foundation doctors/interns).

However, there is as yet no consensus on nomenclature in this area. Peer education is also called peer-assisted learning (PAL), which involves people from similar social groupings who are not professional teachers helping each other to learn and learning themselves by teaching (Topping, 1996). Thus peers are not acting as experts as such, but as colleagues with experiences that the learners will also face in the future.

Near-peer teaching is a form of 'vertical integration', which has also been defined in a variety of ways. One useful, frequently cited definition of vertical integration is that of GPET (General Practice Education and Training in Australia): 'the coordinated, purposeful, planned system of linkages and activities in the delivery of education and training throughout the continuum of the learner's stages of medical education' (GPET, 2003). The learners' stages range from medical school, through prevocational hospital training (i.e. UK foundation posts, internship), vocational/specialist training and on to continuing professional development.

Three dimensions have been suggested to categorise peer teaching: the difference in levels between the learner and teacher; the formality of the interaction; and the number of learners being taught (ten Cate and Durning, 2007a).

Rationale

The principal rationale for peer teaching at medical school is that medical students need to develop skills in education. Doctors spend much of their time communicating with patients, including informing and educating patients about health promotion and disease prevention. They are also involved in facilitating the learning of juniors throughout the continuum of medical education. Thus doctors need to be able to teach and to facilitate learning. Learning outcomes in many curricula and accreditation standards for medical students and doctors in training include those related to education. For example, the General Medical Council (GMC) stipulates that medical graduates should be able to 'communicate effectively in various roles' including teacher (GMC, 2009, p. 22) and 'reflect, learn and teach others' (GMC, 2009, p. 27). The CANMeds 'scholar' role includes being a medical educator and teacher (Frank et al., 2015).

Peer teaching may also help alleviate the teaching burden of faculty members and clinical tutors, as well as enhancing intrinsic motivation; student teachers are motivated to learn the material they are teaching in more depth (ten Cate and Durning, 2007b).

Evidence

One systematic review of peer teaching in the health professions, that included 12 papers, found evidence of mainly positive outcomes (Secomb, 2008). However, this review reported on studies where the focus was peer learning with a clinical tutor, rather than peer teaching as defined above. A later review included 19 papers and concluded that the available evidence suggests many perceived benefits of PAL, though there are concerns about peer assessment and feedback (Burgess et al., 2014). Students who do teach report greater confidence in their teaching ability and presentation skills (Marton et al., 2015) and mentorship skills, organisation, accountability and people management (Secomb, 2008).

Learning and teaching activities

At medical school, the most commonly described activities for peer learning and teaching are anatomy and clinical skills (Marton et al., 2015). Foundation doctors and interns teach through role modelling and having senior students shadow them. They provide support during student assistantships, when students take on increasing responsibility for patient care under supervision to prepare for their own transition into being physicians. The relationship between near peers is obviously less hierarchical and therefore tends to be more relaxed. As with all learning and teaching activities, the learning outcomes need to be defined and known by both learners and teachers (Box 29.1).

Training for the educator role

Doctors are not able to facilitate learning just because they are doctors, though 'doctor' comes from the Latin word to teach, *docere*. While all students and doctors in training should have core training in education, those who wish to take on a more formal role in peer education will need to undertake more extensive learning. This may be during student-selected components, options or electives, or doctors in training may choose to do a clinical fellowship with education responsibilities. Development should include such topics as learning and teaching theories and observed practice; curriculum development; assessment and feedback evaluation.

Peer appraisal of teaching

Within academia, peers are also involved in a number of scholarly activities, including peer review of papers submitted to journals and peer appraisal of teaching. Institutions are beginning to mandate that university teachers undergo an appraisal process periodically that includes having a learning and teaching session observed by a peer, followed by a feedback dialogue. Such peer review has been shown to enhance skills (Regan-Smith et al., 2007). Peer review of medical students and junior doctors undertaking teaching activities should also be in place to help improve their skills.

Various tools guide feedback in relation to teaching and facilitating learning, for example WATCH, the 15-item Warwick Assessment insTrument for Clinical Teaching (Haider et al., 2015) (Box 29.2).

30 Communication

- Communication is important at all levels of healthcare interactions
- Observation of communication during learning activities and patient interactions followed by feedback is absolutely necessary for skills' development
- Role modelling of good communication by all clinical teachers reinforces learning

Box 30.1 Examples of competencies

- Introducing oneself
- Gathering information
- Sharing information
- Exploring ideas, concerns, expectations and effects on life
- Shared decision making
- Used of open and closed questions
- Recognising cues
- Understanding non-verbal cues
- Being empathic and expressing compassion
- Handling emotions
- Telephone and electronic communication
- Written communication
- Accurate documentation
- Open disclosure

Box 30.2 Examples of learning activities

- Watching and appraising video clips of patient–doctor interactions
- Role play with peers
- Working with simulated patients, who give feedback
- Interactions with patients in clinics or community settings to explore their stories and perspectives on health and illness
- Observed (real) patient interactions in clinics
- Interactions in group activities such as problem-based learning

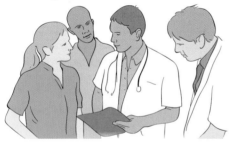

With colleagues

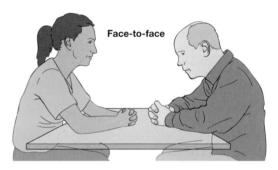

Face-to-face

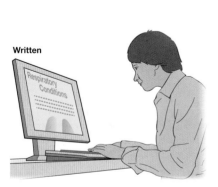

Written

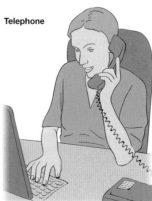

Telephone

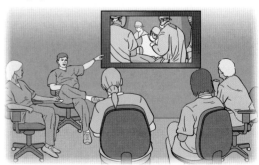

Giving a presentation

Being able to understand one another and be understood are fundamental requirements for the delivery of both education and health care. Communication is important at all levels of practice: between patients and professionals; between healthcare professionals themselves; and between learners and educators. It involves oral and written forms plus verbal and non-verbal skills. Communication skills' training at medical school tends to focus on the patient–doctor interaction, although increasing emphasis is being placed on teamwork and patient handover. The research base relating to communication overwhelmingly indicates that the outcomes of good communication skills include more accurate diagnosis, greater patient satisfaction, improved patient safety and enhanced rates of patient adherence to management plans including prescriptions, as well as greater doctors' well-being (see for example Leonard et al., 2004; Silverman et al., 2005).

Communication and consultation skills should continue to improve over a doctor's career. Feedback from colleagues and patients is important to help professionals review skills, and should be actively sought.

The communication curriculum

In the past, communication competencies were frequently separated from the clinical tasks of history gathering and management planning. This may partially account for the documented deterioration in student communication skills over the medical programme. While the basics of communication may be built upon in the early years of a course, these should not be neglected during clinical teaching. The medical, psychosocial, cultural and spiritual elements of communication should be integrated through the *biopsychosocial model* and a *patient-centred* approach. The communication curriculum is ideally longitudinal and spiral, with students building on previous learning as they advance, without forgetting what has gone before. Tasks become more complex, and communication remains an important element of all learning.

Communication outcomes and competencies

A number of frameworks for communication skills outcomes are available (e.g. Silverman et al., 2005; von Fragstein et al., 2008). These may be broken down into components of communication (with patients and colleagues) and discrete tasks (Box 30.1).

Examples of communication tasks

- Eliciting a history
- Explaining investigations and procedures
- Discussing the meaning of test results
- Discussing management options
- Presenting a patient history
- Obtaining informed consent
- Patient handover
- Writing a discharge and referral letter
- Discussing a patient's condition with another health professional
- Comforting a distressed patient
- Dealing with aggression
- Disclosing an error to a senior colleague
- Working with an interpreter
- Breaking bad news
- Chairing a meeting
- Giving a presentation
- Leading a multidisciplinary team on a task or case conference

---

Learning activities

As with any skill, communication education needs to be experiential and authentic, and appropriate for the level of the learner. Theory needs to be integrated with practice to keep learners motivated (Box 30.2). For rehearsal and enhancement of skills at all level of training and practice, learning with simulated (standardised) patients has been widely adopted (Nestel and Bearman, 2015).

Feedback

A number of structured feedback tools are available. For group work with simulated patients the Calgary–Cambridge Guide (Silverman et al., 2005) is helpful and involves the simulated patient in the debriefing process as an equal partner. It is important to explore the learner's agenda prior and after the learning activity and define the desired learning outcomes. The learner as interviewer should be encouraged to reflect on performance followed by the whole group as active learners. As ever, feedback should be constructive; however, areas for change do need to be identified for learning to occur. Simulation gives learners the chance to replay the scenario and try out processes with which they are unfamiliar in a safe environment. Moreover, anyone in the activity can ask for a pause (or time out) during a scenario to question, clarify or deal with emotions.

Assessment

Communication often forms part of the checklist in Objective Structured Clinical Examination (OSCE) stations. However, communication should not be limited to formal or summative assessment situations. Learners need to be observed regularly interacting with patients in diverse situations. The Mini-Clinical Exercise (mini-CEX) is a work-based assessment tool that may be used for observation, but time for feedback dialogue is required in order for learners to improve (see Chapter 41). Less frequently, unannounced or incognito simulated patients are involved in the assessment of real-life performance in clinics. See Chapters 40–43 for more examples of assessments of communication skills.

Barriers to good communication

All professionals need to be aware of the barriers to good communication and have an awareness of when interactions are becoming dysfunctional. Issues might include power dynamics, cultural differences and physical or sensory impairments. Because learners in clinical situations are often supernumerary, they have plenty of time to elicit histories and interact with patients. In real life, which is mimicked in learning activities and assessments, time pressures contribute to cutting corners and a possible lack of empathy. In particular, doctors in training have to learn to cope with multitasking and prioritising; this may lead to suboptimal patient and colleague interactions, which can be exacerbated by tiredness and stress.

31 Problem-based and case-based learning

Practice points

- Problem-based learning (PBL) and case-based learning (CBL) are inquiry-based learning approaches where learners typically work in small groups around a scenario or case
- The evidence as to effectiveness (whether and why) is unclear
- CBL is evaluated positively by learners and facilitators
- Training for facilitators and orientation for learners are essential

Box 31.1 Definitions

Problem-based learning

'... learning that results from the process of working towards the understanding of a resolution of a problem. The problem is encountered first in the learning process' (Barrows and Tamblyn, 1980, p. 74).

Case-based learning

'...is a learning and teaching approach that aims to prepare students for clinical practice, through the use of authentic clinical cases. These cases link theory to practice, through the application of knowledge to the cases, and encourage the use of inquiry-based learning methods' (Thistlethwaite et al., 2012).

Box 31.2 Role of group and facilitator

PBL model

1. Problem presented to group
2. Group clarifies concepts and terms
3. Questions related to problems defined
4. Learning outcomes set
5. Identification of processes to answer questions and meet learning outcomes
6. Tasks shared out between group members
7. Research solutions
8. Meet consensus on solutions/explanations
9. Revisit learning outcomes.

In **CBL** the case is presented to the group and the learning outcomes are defined by the facilitator.

Both models may involve typically one to three facilitated group meetings, combined with self-directed group and individual work as necessary.

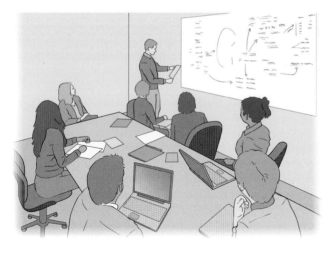

Figure 31.1 Four levels of inquiry-based learning. Source: adapted from Banchi and Bell, 2008.

Confirmation: answers to questions known in advance

Structured: questions, learning outcomes and process provided by facilitator, learners generate explanations
← CBL

Guided: questions & learning outcomes provided by facilitator; learners choose own process to generate explanations
← PBL

Open: learners develop questions, learning outcomes and process to generate explanations

Problem-based learning (PBL) and case-based learning (CBL) are types of learner-centred inquiry-based learning that use whole-task models to facilitate complex learning in groups (though CBL is sometimes an individual pursuit). As the names obviously indicate, CBL broadly speaking involves the use of cases such as patient histories (or journeys) to help meet learning outcomes while PBL focuses on 'problems' or scenarios that may be drawn from a number of sources including patients, communities and workplace relationships. Both approaches embody constructivist theories of education in which learners are encouraged to be active rather than passive participants.

CBL is a long-standing and well-established educational method. The **case method** for teaching pathology, for example, was introduced by James Lorrain Smith in Edinburgh in 1912 with the aim of linking medical students' scientific knowledge with clinical practice (Sturdy, 2007). However, CBL as used in several other disciplines such as law, management and education, comes in many guises and a simple definition is lacking. A best evidence medical education (BEME) systematic review of CBL suggests one definition emphasising the importance of the linkage between theory and practice as its goal (Thistlethwaite *et al.*, 2012b).

PBL was introduced into medical education in the 1960s at McMaster University in Canada, and was widely adopted globally from the 1970s. The original McMaster model, taken up by Maastricht University and used widely internationally, has since been modified over the years, although common elements of PBL include the use of trigger materials to stimulate group discussion and learning, with the possibility of more than one solution to any problem.

One main difference between traditional PBL and CBL is that students define their own learning outcomes for the former whereas for the latter the outcomes are presented by the facilitator. Thus PBL is typically less structured than CBL, which some learners may find disconcerting (Srinivasan *et al.*, 2007). Learner orientation to both methods is required, as well as facilitator training and professional development.

Evidence for effectiveness

As with many curricular developments in medical education, it is difficult to prove direct cause and effect between interventions and learning. In relation to CBL, the BEME review (Thistlethwaite *et al.,* 2012b) included 104 papers relating to health professional education. The main findings included that CBL:

• Most frequently involves small face-to-face groups (two to 15 learners) but groups are sometimes large with more than 30
• May be delivered online
• Can be introduced through a lecture but then involves interaction between learners
• Is evaluated positively by learners and facilitators
• Appears to promote learning but there is little evidence it is more effective than other educational methods
• Helps link biomedical sciences to real-life patient presentations by enhancing relevance and understanding of concepts.

Papers published since the BEME review also highlight the need to prepare learners and faculty for CBL, and to ensure that facilitators do not overly intervene in the learning process (Thistlethwaite, 2015c).

A number of studies and reviews of PBL have been carried out over the years, which have had conflicting results (O'Brien, 2015). In particular, according to some critics, the outcomes of PBL compared to other learning approaches are not sufficiently better to justify the extra resources required for this labour-intensive process (O'Brien, 2015). Many medical schools have increased group size and reduced facilitation time to cut costs, raising further questions about what should be regarded as 'true' PBL.

Implementation

PBL and CBL require learning materials: problems, cases and learner and teacher guides. These should be tailored to match the learning outcomes at specific points of the overall programme. Problems and cases should encourage deep learning, building on prior knowledge and be authentic. Writing takes time and each problem/case will need input and feedback from suitable content experts working together to integrate learning. Facilitator and learner guides are important and ongoing evaluation is necessary to keep material up-to-date, relevant and interesting. Clinical colleagues are good sources of patient stories and supporting documentation such as de-identified imaging and blood test results.

Each small group (however this is defined at an institution) needs a facilitator – someone who is an expert in process and not necessarily in content. While students like to have clinicians involved with their group, this is not always possible. In CBL a flipped classroom approach may be useful: learners are given the case to work on before the formal session so they can come prepared with background reading. Ideally, learners should work in their groups with minimal input from the facilitator, who should however be prepared to intervene when necessary to move the group on. Novice facilitators need to be trained and supported by a peer until they feel ready to work on their own. A poor facilitator can be very destructive to a group. In addition, first year students, who may be unfamiliar with small group and student-centred learning, need sufficient orientation to the method and expectations.

Assessment

Frequently, the performance of learners and their team-working skills during PBL and CBL discussions are assessed. This may be through facilitator observation and grading, or peer review. Assessment will usually focus on group-working skills, application, professionalism, problem solving and clinical reasoning. Consideration has to be given to how this may affect learning and group dynamics. There may be tensions between the role of facilitator and role of assessor. Timing and quantity of assessment should not be onerous. Remediation should be in place for those who perform unsatisfactorily.

32 Learner support

Practice points

- Medical students and doctors in training can require extra support academically, pastorally and in the development of coping strategies for clinical practice
- A successful support system has multiple access points and integrates support within the curriculum or learning environment
- Those involved in learner support must be trained to recognise the signs of a struggler and have knowledge of referral processes
- Occasionally, learners are not suitable for a medical career and, then, support should shift to alternative careers' guidance

Clinical placement lead
Placement administration lead
Clinical support tutor
Placement teaching staff
Placement administration team
Student support system
Course teaching staff
Course administration team
Personal tutor
Course lead
Course administration lead

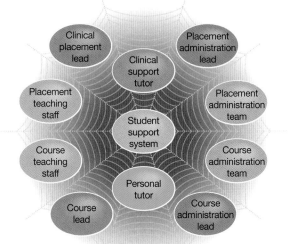

Figure 32.1 The 'web of support' for undergraduate students. A good support system should have multiple access points, with all recognised front-line staff trained in referral processes that direct the learner into the support system, whether the student is on clinical placement or university based. Source: Vogan *et al.*, 2013.

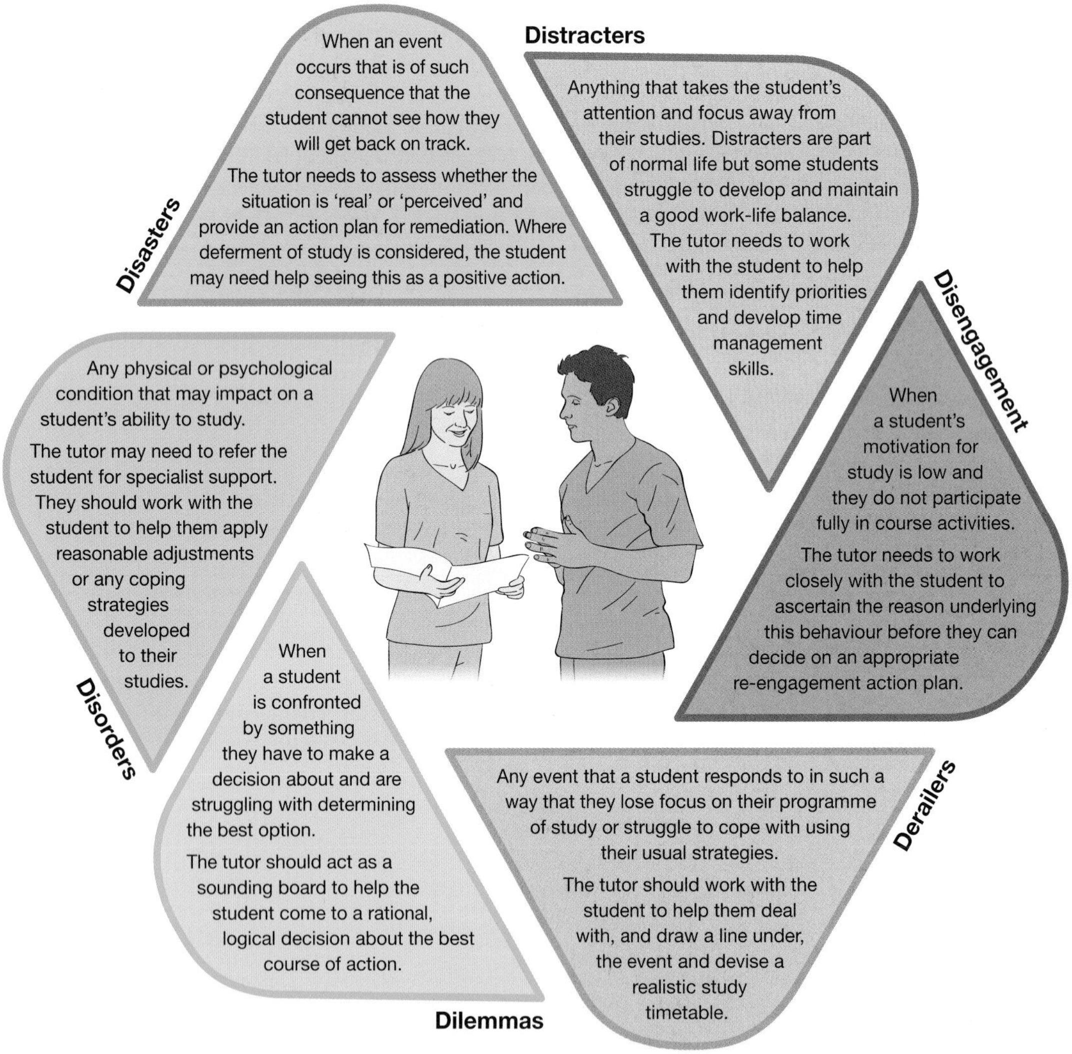

Disasters
When an event occurs that is of such consequence that the student cannot see how they will get back on track.
The tutor needs to assess whether the situation is 'real' or 'perceived' and provide an action plan for remediation. Where deferment of study is considered, the student may need help seeing this as a positive action.
Distracters
Anything that takes the student's attention and focus away from their studies. Distracters are part of normal life but some students struggle to develop and maintain a good work-life balance.
The tutor needs to work with the student to help them identify priorities and develop time management skills.
Disengagement
When a student's motivation for study is low and they do not participate fully in course activities.
The tutor needs to work closely with the student to ascertain the reason underlying this behaviour before they can decide on an appropriate re-engagement action plan.
Derailers
Any event that a student responds to in such a way that they lose focus on their programme of study or struggle to cope with using their usual strategies.
The tutor should work with the student to help them deal with, and draw a line under, the event and devise a realistic study timetable.
Dilemmas
When a student is confronted by something they have to make a decision about and are struggling with determining the best option.
The tutor should act as a sounding board to help the student come to a rational, logical decision about the best course of action.
Disorders
Any physical or psychological condition that may impact on a student's ability to study.
The tutor may need to refer the student for specialist support. They should work with the student to help them apply reasonable adjustments or any coping strategies developed to their studies.

Figure 32.2 The Swansea Six Ds Model. A framework developed at Swansea University Medical School to be used by those involved in identifying and helping students in difficulty. It provides a lens through which student difficulties can be visualised and managed by a support tutor. The complete tool (not shown) takes each of the six 'Ds' and describes what might be going on for the student, outlines some positive and negative aspects associated with the descriptor and suggests referral and remediation strategies. Source: Vogan *et al.*, 2014.

The journey through medical education and training can be a complicated pathway and, although they may not always realise it, even the most talented, independent people need guidance to successfully navigate their way through. At various points along the way, all learners need signposting in order to complete their journey safely, some need additional help. Thus, any learner support system should be designed in such a way that it can cater for the needs of all, whilst being flexible enough to be tailored to the requirements of individuals. The role and degree of involvement of medical educators within the learner support system is varied, but the aim is to enable as many students and doctors in training as possible to complete their journey safely and have successful clinical careers.

Extra support may be required

Learners at all stages can potentially require extra support in a range of areas, whether they are based at a university or in the clinical or healthcare environment. Firstly, learners can struggle with the academic content at any stage of training and an inability to address serious academic issues can often result in the learner failing to progress to the next stage of training. Tackling academic struggles effectively usually requires an individualised programme with specialist input. Secondly, pastoral support can help deal with a range of difficulties that may have an impact on a learner's performance and are often, but not always, linked to circumstances outside training. Such difficulties can include making the transition to university life or postgraduate training, financial or career planning, developing a good work-life balance and dealing with situations that arise in their personal lives, for example bereavement. Lastly, learners may have been assessed as having a disability that requires help with the development of coping strategies or the implementation of reasonable adjustments to the learning and/or clinical environment. At the undergraduate level, university student support services are usually well-equipped to deal with any disability-linked difficulties encountered in university life or on clinical placements, including specialist support and advice. Similarly, in addition to occupational health, doctors in training will usually have access to services that can give specialist support and tuition linked to their disability. At any point in training, learners may also develop either short or long-term illnesses or have accidents that may require either temporary or permanent modifications to their learning environment. Once again, specialist support and advice can often be sorted out through the university student support services and/or occupational health.

An integrated, supportive approach

Medicine programmes are professionally accredited and have fitness to practice requirements, so it is vital that the learning environment is one where learners feel free to disclose and discuss any problems that may potentially affect their studies. Medical students (and qualified doctors) are often scared and unsure about fitness to practice and believe that declaration of even minor struggles will have a detrimental effect on their current studies and future careers (Chew-Graham et al., 2003).

Overcoming these barriers can be challenging but having a support system with multiple access points (Figure 32.1) means that learners can easily access help wherever they are based and are more likely to find someone they feel comfortable talking to. Often, rather than referring on, the person to whom the struggler first presents takes on too much of the burden of supporting that learner (see the Six Ds model (Figure 32.2) for ideas around 'diagnosing' what is going on for the learner). When dealing with a learner needing specialised support, it is important to understand the limits of your expertise and role boundaries and to know about existing specialist support services. This is particularly important for clinical teachers, as referral processes for students are likely to be different from those used for patients or doctors in training.

An inclusive learning environment

Both medical students and doctors in training are particularly vulnerable to health issues such as anxiety, depression, stress and burnout (e.g. Dyrbye et al., 2006, 2014). A number of professional bodies (e.g. in the UK the Medical Schools' Council, and General Medical Council, 2015; Department of Health, 2008) suggest that undergraduate curriculum planning needs to incorporate elements that enable all students to develop effective coping strategies to deal with the pressures of a career in medicine, and all students should be encouraged to maintain a healthy level of extracurricular activities (Kjeldstadli et al., 2006). Support staff and tutors need to be mindful of particularly stressful times for their learners (e.g. in the run-up to and during exams, early or psychologically challenging clinical rotations) and be proactive in these periods with the inclusion of suitable support and debriefing activities. Curricular design and teaching sessions should be inclusive to all and, if possible, have some degree of flexibility and/or sympathetic timetabling to accommodate those with short-term illnesses, ethnic or religious considerations or specialist support requirements.

Identify struggling learners early

Particularly amongst large undergraduate cohorts, strugglers can often go unnoticed until they start failing assignments, have serious performance issues or have reached crisis point. Ideally, all programmes should have mechanisms by which they can identify strugglers or learners who have the potential to develop difficulties early and put support in place before the assessment burden becomes too great or a student reaches the point where the only realistic option is to suspend or withdraw. All those that are in regular contact with the learner should be provided with training and frameworks to help them identify and deal with learners in difficulty (e.g. Hicks et al., 2005; Hays et al., 2011; Yates, 2011). They should be proactive in feeding back worries or concerns about individual learners to those in charge of the training and support system, and be reassured that this information with be dealt with sympathetically and confidentially.

A duty of care

Whilst we do have a duty of care to ensure learners are fully supported and given every opportunity to succeed, we should not forget that we also have a duty of care to their current and future patients. Making the decision that a career in medicine is not the right pathway can be difficult for learners and those who support them, particularly for those that are heavily involved in the support. Research suggests that clinical teachers are often reluctant to fail learners in practice (Cleland et al., 2008), thus having structures where decisions about failures of assessment and fitness to practice are independent from those who are heavily involved in the support system is particularly important. In cases where learners are potentially leaving medicine, the support offered should also include alternative careers' guidance.

33 Supporting professional development activities

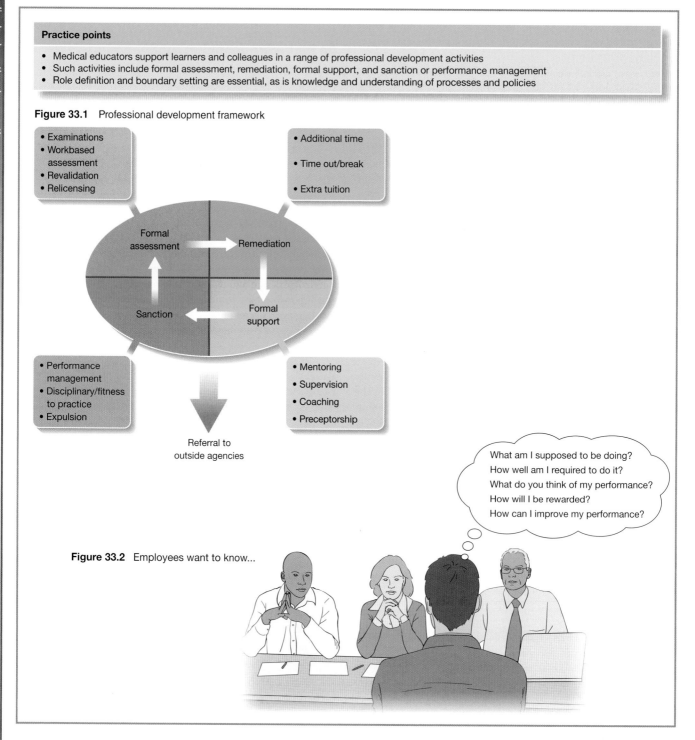

Figure 33.1 Professional development framework

- Examinations
- Workbased assessment
- Revalidation
- Relicensing

- Additional time
- Time out/break
- Extra tuition

Formal assessment → Remediation

Sanction ← Formal support

- Performance management
- Disciplinary/fitness to practice
- Expulsion

- Mentoring
- Supervision
- Coaching
- Preceptorship

Referral to outside agencies

What am I supposed to be doing?
How well am I required to do it?
What do you think of my performance?
How will I be rewarded?
How can I improve my performance?

Figure 33.2 Employees want to know...

All health professionals are required to engage in professional development activities of some kind, including attending courses and conferences, reading, updating and undertaking mandatory training. This chapter considers professional development from the perspective of the person providing it, rather than who is undertaking it (Chapter 45 looks at how educators might engage in professional development themselves). It also explores strategies that may have to be used when an individual's performance falls below expected standards.

Many professional development and learner support activities are very similar in the skills and knowledge required by educators (see Chapters 32 and 34), but some differences in approach, process and outcome are useful to understand. At certain stages of career, particularly at times of transition, organisations provide different modes of professional development and support and it is helpful to understand these to enable others to reach their potential and develop their own practice. Whether you are involved in supervision, appraisal, mentoring or formal assessment, the foundations of developing good relationships and communicating well are fundamental.

A professional development framework

When considering how best to engage with students, doctors in training, peers or other colleagues in professional development (or performance management) activities, it is essential to define your exact role, what will be expected from you in terms of time commitment, activities and duration of the relationship. Figure 33.1 sets out some of the key elements involved in professional development activities, each of which needs a different skill set and role definition.

The framework can be used to consider what help or support an individual might need at different stages of their training or career or when making a transition to a new role or job. From the top left, you can see that **formal assessment** can be ongoing throughout an individual's working life, not only in terms of professional examinations or assignments in postgraduate study, but also relating to relicensing or revalidation requirements or workplace based assessments, such as 360 degree appraisals, case discussions or Mini-Clinical Exercises (mini-CEX). Teachers and clinicians have a huge role in assessing learners, in the university setting, in clinical practice and for national examinations. Depending on the nature of the assessment, you may be required to give formal written or verbal feedback on knowledge and understanding, practical skills and/or professional behaviours. Understanding how to give meaningful, constructive feedback is essential if you are to help learners develop as competent, safe, caring practitioners (see Chapter 37).

Moving clockwise round the framework, sometimes a form of **remediation** may be needed to help support a struggling or failing individual. In formal assessments, learners with a defined learning disability (such as dyslexia or dyspraxia) may be entitled to extra time in written assessments or to use spell-checkers in clinical practice. Depending on your role, you may be asked to provide additional tutorials or to give specific support and feedback to those who are struggling, perhaps with clinical procedures or communication skills. For individuals with more complicated health or personal problems, time out may be either a necessity (e.g. with a physical or mental health problem) or a useful strategy to enable someone to get back on track.

Formal support can be carried out in a number of ways. In university settings, academic support may be provided by tutors in the subject and personal support by pastoral or personal tutors. These roles are usually fairly well separated so as to enable students to receive more objective assessments and to be able to share worries and concerns with someone who can help them.

Finally, some individuals may need to receive a form of **sanction**. This might be for academic failure, in which case remediation might be offered up to a point, but ultimately failure will lead to expulsion or failure to progress. For unprofessional behaviours (either in education/training or in the workplace) sanctions might include performance management, disciplinary procedures or fitness to practice procedures for serious cases (Vogan *et al.*, 2014a), see also Chapters 28, 32 and 42.

For many issues, it is often helpful to have knowledge of outside referral agencies and what they can provide. These include wellbeing or counselling provision; occupational health and external organisations such as Alcoholics Anonymous. Underpinning all these activities are formal processes, policies and procedures which serve to protect the individuals involved, the organisation, the profession and patients. Ultimately, patient safety is the driving force behind all types of professional development, support and sanction.

Appraisal

Practising professionals (and increasingly students) are required to engage in regular appraisal. Appraisal (sometimes called performance review) is a formal process designed to measure how well a person is meeting defined goals and objectives, which are themselves aligned with organisational and/or professional objectives. The specific purpose and scope of appraisal varies between professions and organisations, but should ideally be appraisee-led, that is the person being appraised defines their objectives, works towards them and provides evidence of achievement. Appraisal is formalised through completion of documentation or computer-based systems. In some instances, appraisal is linked to revalidation or relicensing.

Coaching

Coaching typically refers to methods of helping others to improve, develop, learn new skills, find personal success, achieve aims and to manage life change and personal challenges. Coaching commonly addresses attitudes, behaviours and knowledge, as well as skills, and can also focus on physical and spiritual development.

www.businessballs.com/coaching.htm.

Coaching therefore aims to develop individual capabilities and potential to unlock performance and achieve personal and/ or organisational goals. Some professional development activities, particularly at senior level, use executive coaching as a means to help develop leadership and management skills and manage transitions. Coaching can be very helpful for people who are at a career crossroads or who need help in making life and work decisions

Mentoring and supervision

Mentors provide guidance, support and sometimes advice for their mentees to help them make transition or change or to assist with their professional development. These may comprise formal or informal roles. Professional, clinical or educational supervision involves formally overseeing performance, giving feedback and supporting professional development (see Chapter 34 for more on these topics).

Counselling

Counselling and psychotherapy are umbrella terms that cover a range of talking therapies. They are delivered by trained practitioners who work with people over a short or long term to help them bring about effective change or enhance their wellbeing.

British Association of Counselling and Psychotherapy definition: www.bacp.co.uk/crs/Training/whatiscounselling.php.

Whilst counselling should always be carried out by trained counsellor, and you need to know when someone might need to be referred, basic counselling skills such as active listening, building rapport and reframing are all useful communication skills that can be used in a range of professional development settings.

34 Mentoring and supervision

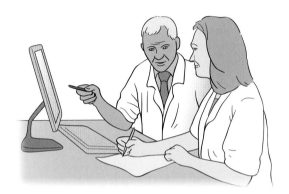

Figure 34.1 The GROW model. Source: www.mentoringforchange.co.uk/classic/ (accessed Sept. 2016). Reproduced with permission of Dr Mike Munro Turner.

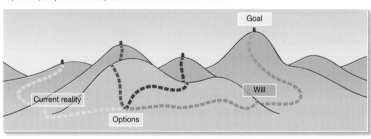

Figure 34.2 Heron's (1986) six categories of interventions

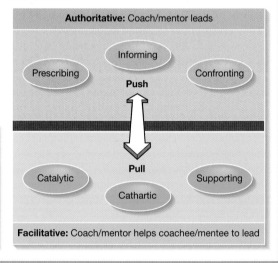

A wide range of individuals provide formal support for learners and colleagues. In this chapter, we look at mentoring and supervision as two of the key activities in which medical educators are often involved. Chapter 33 provides more detail about other activities with which educators may be involved in supporting others' professional development activities. It also introduces a framework to help select the right activity for different roles, (see Figure 33.1) which is also relevant to mentoring and supervision.

Building relationships

Building an effective relationship is central, which involves mutual respect, trust and a willingness to engage in the process. Both mentoring and supervision require effective communication in a safe physical and psychological environment. This is particularly important when discussing personal or difficult issues or giving negative feedback. It is the responsibility of the mentor or supervisor to limit barriers to communication including physical barriers (e.g. disruptive environment; language); psychosocial barriers (e.g. anxiety; fear or authority) or professional barriers (e.g. lack of knowledge; power imbalance).

Mentoring

Mentors provide guidance, support and sometimes advice for the benefit of the mentee to help make transition or change or to assist professional development. Sometimes called 'the guide on the side' or a 'wise counsel', a mentor is typically more senior or more experienced than the mentee. The benefits for mentees include improved performance and productivity; career opportunities and advancement; improved knowledge and skills; and greater confidence and wellbeing (Garvey and Garrett-Harris, 2005).

What people want from a mentor

- Professional credibility
- Knows the organisation well
- A positive, supportive role model who motivates and guides
- Willingness to invest in the mentee, give time and share expertise and knowledge
- Willing to challenge and push when needed
- Sets clear boundaries
- Provides good advice
- Maintains professional confidentiality
- Is trustworthy

Medical Education at a Glance, First Edition. Edited by Judy McKimm, Kirsty Forrest and Jill Thistlethwaite © 2017 John Wiley & Sons, Ltd. Published 2017 by John Wiley & Sons, Ltd.

Many organisations have formal mentoring schemes for new staff to help them in their new job. The benefits to the organisation include increased motivation and performance; policy implementation; better 'talent' management; enhanced knowledge and skills; support for change initiatives and active succession planning. Some schemes also use peer mentoring, where people of a similar stage and career level mentor one another.

Mentoring models

A number of models exist that have been designed to support mentors and mentees, which are also useful in coaching, supervision and personal tutoring. Clutterbuck (2004) suggests two main models:
- The **sponsorship** model: where a mentor takes on a protégé, the mentor has power and influence and can help the mentee achieve organisational or professional goals.
- The **developmental** model: helps the mentee find their own solutions – this has longer-term sustainability and often fits into a formal organisational or professional scheme.

The GROW model (Figure 34.1)

This model provides a simple framework to helping the mentee work towards their goal (Whitmore, 2009). It can be used in a number of ways, but the idea behind it is that when setting **G**oals, it is useful to start with the current **R**eality or to set some provisional goals, then come back to the current reality to generate **O**ptions. When thinking about the current reality, some difficult conversations may result, which may be about **W**ill, that is motivation, willingness to develop and, sometimes, to change.

Heron's categories of interventions (Figure 34.2)

Heron's (1986) model looks at six interventions, broadly categorised into those that the mentor leads (more authoritative) and those that are primarily led by the mentee, where the mentor is more facilitative. The mentor needs to choose their approach and tactics carefully in response to the situation or needs of the individual.

The more authoritative interventions (where you are trying to *push* the person into action or changing behaviours) include:

Prescribing: here you may ask or require or strongly suggest that the individual does something.
Informing: this may be about responding to a request or providing some factual information.
Confronting: confronting can be telling the individual something they may not want to hear, perhaps based on some feedback from other people. Or it can be 'in the moment', for example if someone contradicts themselves, makes unrealistic assumptions about their skills and aspirations or challenges your role or credibility.

The more facilitative approaches aim to help (*pull*) the person to develop and find solutions for themselves, they include:

Catalytic: here you are trying to provide a stimulus for action and development and provide motivation and inspiration so that the person feels they have the inner resources to take steps towards development.

Cathartic: in this approach you are providing a safe place for someone to discuss difficult or emotional experiences, or to speak about situations they are struggling with.

You may use counselling skills such as active listening, reflecting and summarising, but you are *not* a counsellor in an education setting. If you think someone needs counselling then you might suggest that would be helpful and provide information about services. Set some time boundaries around cathartic conversations, so that the person moves into an 'adult' goal-setting mode before the meeting finishes.

Supporting: might be through a number of ways such as responding to their development needs, being at the end of the phone in times when they are having difficulties or giving advice when asked.

Supervision

Professional, clinical or educational supervision involves overseeing performance, giving feedback and supporting professional development. Supervisors in medical education have a specific role and defined responsibilities within postgraduate training. In many professions, ongoing supervision is required for professionals to continue practising. Supervision usually involves a close relationship in which difficult or challenging cases are discussed or professional practice is developed. Effective supervision has been demonstrated to improve clinical practice and patient outcomes (Kilminster et al., 2000).

Supervision is about:

Cases/events/situations: ethical issues, complex decision making, difficult interpersonal situations, complaints or other significant events
Contexts: teamworking, professional or interprofessional issues, role or boundary conflict, communication problems
Careers: training needs, future plans, work conditions, managing and delegating work.

A range of techniques and approaches can be used in both informal and formal settings, for brief interventions and for long-term relationships. Whilst much professional development is carried out on a one-to-one basis, some development activities are carried out in groups. These include action learning sets, step back groups, group supervision meetings and tutorials. Good communication skills, relationship building and understanding both your own role and those of your mentee or supervisee are essential. Being able to set clear goals, action plans and ensure follow-up activities is central to supporting the person with whom you are working to achieve success. In addition, you need to be able to provide additional support when needed, know when to refer to other agencies or individuals and know the boundaries of both your roles. Keeping good documentation is important, particularly if you are working in a remedial or disciplinary role, although it shouldn't be onerous and distract you from conversations.

35 e-Learning

Figure 35.1 The e-learning spectrum

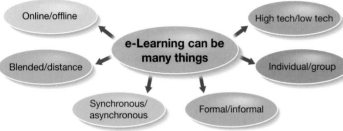

Figure 35.2 The e-learning toolbox

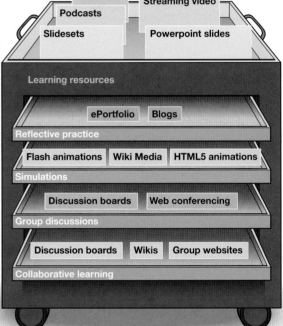

Box 35.1 Pros and cons of e-learning

Cons

- High development overheads
- Server to maintain?
- Staff training/support
- Potential for student isolation

Pros

- Study anytime, anywhere
- Facilitates group work and collaboration
- New disruptive approaches possible
- Utilisation of mobile devices
- Economy of scale
- Re-use of matrerials
- Interactivity

Table 35.1 Modes of delivery

	Physical presence of tutor	Virtual presence of tutor	Electronically delivered content	Synchronous electronic communication	Asynchronous electronic communication
Face-to-face	✓				
Technology enhanced face-to-face	✓		✓	✓	
Self-directed learning			✓		
Distance learning (asynchronous)		✓	✓		✓
Distance learning (synchronous)		✓	✓	✓	
Blended/hybrid (asynchronous)	✓	✓	✓		✓
Blended/hybrid (synchronous)	✓	✓	✓	✓	

The term 'e-learning' describes the use of electronic media and/or technology with the aim to improve the effectiveness of the learning process. Historically, e-learning was made available via computer terminals in university laboratories or on media such as DVD. Now e-learning is delivered mostly via the internet so the term 'online learning' is also often used, although it can take many forms (Figure 35.1). The degree to which e-learning may replace other, more traditional methodologies within a programme varies on a continuum from none to a fully online distance learning course.

Advantages and challenges

e-Learning has many advantages for the learner, but perhaps the most significant is encapsulated in the phrase 'anytime, anyplace'. Material can be revisited, perused at varying speeds and include self-assessment. The teacher has the ability to teach large groups over a wide geographical area. However, e-learning is not cost free, as the design, delivery and maintenance of e-learning programmes need initial capital and further resources. See Box 35.1 for some of the benefits and challenges of e-learning.

How to design an e-learning module

When embarking on the development of e-learning material, the first question to be asked is: 'is e-learning the right solution?' In order to answer this question, the following questions will need to be considered:

- What is expected of the online course?
- Will it replace or supplement existing teaching?
- Is an online course the best choice?
- What will the costs be and who will maintain and update the course?
- Who will finally approve the course? What are their expectations?
  The needs analysis should also include a user analysis:
- Who are the target learners?
- Will they be able to access the course site and perform all the necessary interactions?
- How will learners benefit from the online course?
- How can learners' progress be evaluated?
  And finally, these are the ideal characteristics that a teacher needs to develop e-learning materials:
- Knowledge of adult learning theory
- Instructional design competence and knowledge of different e-learning solutions
- Skills to use the e-learning development software tool
- An awareness of basic graphic design principles
- The skills to manipulate images in a graphic design software tool.
  However, many teachers are too busy to become proficient in the use of authoring tools such as Dreamweaver™. Often, Internet designers will do the authoring; however, when writing the material bearing in mind the way it will be viewed and presented is vital. Also, the education basics should not be lost: having educational goals, providing the learning, assessing lessons learned and providing feedback.

Design considerations

Often, you will be adapting material you already have – previous lectures or book chapters – but it is highly likely that such materials will have to be rewritten for course content on the web. Keep the language simple and friendly, especially if there is no teacher contact to provide the human touch. Content needs to be presented in an engaging and non-threatening way. Incorporate motivational elements such as certificates on completion and discussion boards

for interaction with other learners. Prepare a flow chart or story board showing how the course progresses from start to finish. The pages containing the course material should be organised in a way that makes navigation easy and simple

Modes of delivery

e-Learning can be described in terms of the delivery mode chosen (Table 35.1). An important distinction is whether teaching is delivered to all students simultaneously or not.

Synchronous delivery is where learning takes place with all learners at the same time as in a traditional face-to-face lecture. An electronic equivalent could be a webinar whereby a teacher broadcasts a teaching session to the group using a web-conferencing system. Most systems allow for some interaction from students, whether text or speech based, in a similar manner to the physical lecture theatre. There are clear benefits of electronic delivery, not least the capacity for the student to 'attend' from wherever they happen to be, although issues such as time zones need to be taken into account.

Asynchronous learning does not occur at the same time or place. In many ways this is a more convenient form of e-learning for a busy professional as it allows them to choose a convenient time to engage. The term encompasses a wide range of learning interactions from discussion boards to learning resources.

Blended learning includes both face-to-face interaction and online learning, leveraging the strengths of each. This has further led to the concept of the flipped classroom, whereby the main bulk of the topic content is delivered via e-learning with face-to-face time reserved for tutorial style discussion around the more complex concepts emerging from the learning materials. Table 35.1 details the distinct modes of blended learning based on whether the e-learning element is delivered synchronously or not.

Learning environments

A virtual learning environment (VLE) or learning management system (LMS) is a platform used for the delivery of e-learning. A number of VLEs are currently used in medical education, for example Moodle™ and Blackboard™. Many VLEs are modelled on traditional face-to-face learning environments and so provide learners with access to teaching materials, tests, assessments etc. They also include social spaces, allowing interaction with both the teacher and other learners. Individual learner accounts are central to the concept of the VLE, allowing progress to be accurately tracked by both the individual and their teacher, thus facilitating feedback from one to the other.

A good VLE will provide most if not all of the tools displayed in Figure 35.2 The tools from our imaginary toolbox are used by the tutor and/or learning technologist to develop a course appropriate to the predetermined delivery model, they become the components of the course. The toolbox metaphor indicates that these tools are readily available, often with minimal effort and are can be selected as necessary. The specific components chosen will very much depend on the nature of the course and should be carefully chosen to align with learning outcomes. So, for example, a content-led course would principally use the tools for learning resources supplemented with other components. On the other hand a learner-led collaborative style course would make greater use of social spaces and media (see Chapter 36). Whatever delivery mode is chosen, good practice dictates that learner-centred active learning should be adopted and that a wide range of activities are included to facilitate engagement and interaction.

36 Social media

Figure 36.1 The seven Cs of social media

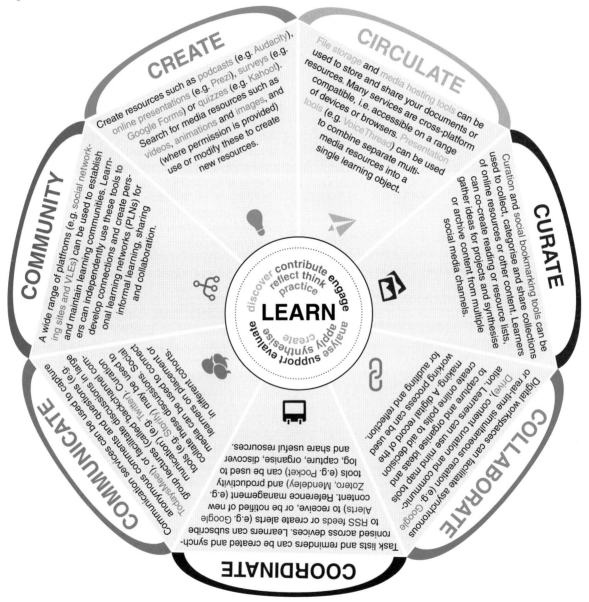

CREATE
Create resources such as podcasts (e.g. Audacity), online presentations (e.g. Prezi), surveys (e.g. Google Forms) or quizzes (e.g. Kahoot). Search for media resources such as videos, animations and images, and (where permission is provided) use or modify these to create new resources.

CIRCULATE
File storage and media hosting tools can be used to store and share your documents or resources. Many services are cross-platform compatible, i.e. accessible on a range of devices or browsers. Presentation tools (e.g. VoiceThread) can be used to combine separate multimedia resources into a single learning object.

CURATE
Curation and social bookmarking tools can be used to collect, categorise and share collections of online resources or other content. Learners can co-create reading or resource lists, gather ideas for projects and synthesise or archive content from multiple social media channels.

COLLABORATE
Digital workspaces can facilitate asynchronous or real-time simultaneous creation and communication (e.g. Google Drive). Learners can use mind map tools to create online polls to aid decision making. A digital record of the working process can be used for auditing and reflection.

COORDINATE
Task lists and reminders can be created and synchronised across devices. Learners can subscribe to RSS feeds or create alerts (e.g. Google Alerts) to receive, or be notified of new content. Reference management (e.g. Zotero, Mendeley) and productivity tools (e.g. Pocket) can be used to log, capture, organise, discover and share useful resources.

COMMUNICATE
Communication services can be used to capture group lectures (facilitate discussions and questions in large lectures) or facilitate backchannel communication) (e.g. Today'sMeet) (e.g. Storify) may be used to collate these discussions. Social media can be used on placements to connect learners in different cohorts.

COMMUNITY
A wide range of platforms (e.g. social networking sites and VLEs) can be used to establish and maintain learning communities. Learners can independently use these tools to develop connections and create personal learning networks (PLNs) for informal learning, sharing and collaboration.

LEARN
discover contribute engage reflect think practice analyse apply synthesise create support evaluate

Table 36.1 Examples of social media tools

Blog	An online web log or journal, e.g. WordPress, Blogger, Weebly, Tumblr	Micro blog	Service for sending short messages or multimedia content, e.g. Twitter, Tumblr
Chart/ diagram tools	Tools to create and share mind maps, charts and other diagrams, e.g. Mindmup, Coggle	Presentation tools	Create and publish online presentations, e.g. Prezi, SlideShare, VoiceThread, Haiku Deck
Collaboration tools	A broad category of tools to facilitate or support collaborative working, e.g. Slack, Trello	RSS readers	Application that aggregates syndicated web content such as news articles, e.g. Feedly, Digg
Curation tools	Create and share collections of online resources or content, e.g. Pinterest, Scoop.it, Storify	Social bookmarking	A tool to collate, tag, comment on and share links to online resources, e.g. Diigo, Delicious
Discussion forums	A platform for posting messages and media content, e.g. Doctors.net, doc2doc.	Social networking	Platform to connect, communicate and share with an online network, e.g. Facebook, Google+
File storage	A service to organise and share files, e.g. Dropbox, Google Drive, OneDrive	Wiki	An online space that can be edited by multiple authors, e.g. Wikipedia, Wikispaces, PBWorks
Media hosting	Store and share audio, animations, images or video content, e.g. Instagram, You Tube, Vimeo	Writing tools	Application for creating or cocreating documents, e.g. Evernote, Google Drive, OneNote

Social media is a broad term used to describe a wide range of online platforms, tools, applications and services that enable users to produce, consume and share content (also referred to as Web 2.0 technologies). Examples of the various types of social media tools are listed in Table 36.1, a number of which can be used free of charge. Many of these technologies and tools are available on virtual learning environment and e-portfolio platforms. Institutions may purchase systems (such as media streaming servers) or install open source systems (e.g. WordPressTM and ElggTM) so that they can be managed, maintained, customised and restricted to only their members.

How is social media being used for learning and teaching?

Social media tools can support social and constructivist forms of teaching and learning (see Chapter 4). The Seven Cs described in Figure 36.1 illustrate a range of activities that can be used by medical educators and/or learners to facilitate and support learning and assessment. Social media technologies are being used in, and in combination with, face-to-face teaching (sometimes referred to as a 'blended' approach), in clinical teaching, to support independent learning and distance learning. These technologies can also support informal learning and CPD activities, and provide opportunities for learners to develop digital capabilities. Case studies and evaluations are widely available online (see Further Reading).

Social media has contributed to the growth of user-generated content and open educational resources (OERs). Definitions of the term OER vary, although generally it is a term applied to resources that are freely available for educational use (Jisc, 2010). However, not all resources accessible online are OERs, and care must be taken to ensure use complies with copyright and other legal requirements (see Jisc, 2010 for further information). OERs can include digital stories, e-books, podcasts, interactive learning objects and multimedia content. FOAM (Free Open-Access Medical education) is a collection of open educational resources, which are created and published predominantly on social media platforms (Nickson and Cadogan, 2014).

Selecting and implementing social media technologies

The latest technological trends and developments can appear tempting. However, as illustrated in Figure 36.1, the learning process should be central to these decisions. Technologies should be selected and implemented in accordance with the intended learning outcomes and learners' needs. Only after these have been determined will it be possible to define the technical and functional requirements. For example, if the learner is required to access the tool in a clinical setting, firewall restrictions and clinical responsibilities need to be considered. It is important to address potential technical issues and devise appropriate mitigation strategies, for example if the service becomes temporarily unavailable or is discontinued. Educators should ensure that they do not exclude learners by making assumptions about their device ownership, preferences, accessibility requirements and digital capabilities. Technical support and training may be required. Your organisation may have guidelines or policies that may restrict the use of third-party technologies.

Managing risks and limitations

Social media technologies raise a number of concerns with regards to anonymity, privacy, confidentiality and data protection. A social media policy should be made available, which clearly outlines potential risks (for the learners and the organisation), acceptable use guidelines and how infringements will be managed. The code of conduct should inform learners of their responsibilities (e.g. to be respectful, maintain confidentiality and professional boundaries). The document may also specify other applicable policies and guidelines such as the UK General Medical Council's guidance document on doctors' use of social media (GMC, 2013a).

Educators need to consider what data will be required, collected and stored by third party social media providers, and whether this adheres to ethical and legal policies. Learners should be aware of the terms when registering for third-party systems, the potential risks of posting online and what privacy controls are provided. They should also be made aware that privacy controls offer limited protection and that privacy cannot be guaranteed. An alternative should be offered to learners who do not agree to the terms or who do not wish to have an account or public profile.

Learners should be informed about the purpose and rationale of the learning activities and chosen technologies. Expectations regarding frequency and modes of engagement should be clarified, with details of how participation will be monitored or assessed if applicable. Educators need to communicate what role they will have in these online spaces, and to what extent they will be participating in discussions. Facilitators or moderators may be required to intervene if conversations go off topic, if learners become distracted or lack motivation. If social media sites are to be used for summative assessment tasks, educators need to consider if the tool can provide a sufficient audit trail on submissions, how unfair practice can be identified and how feedback will be provided. Personal academic feedback disseminated on social media sites may violate learners' privacy.

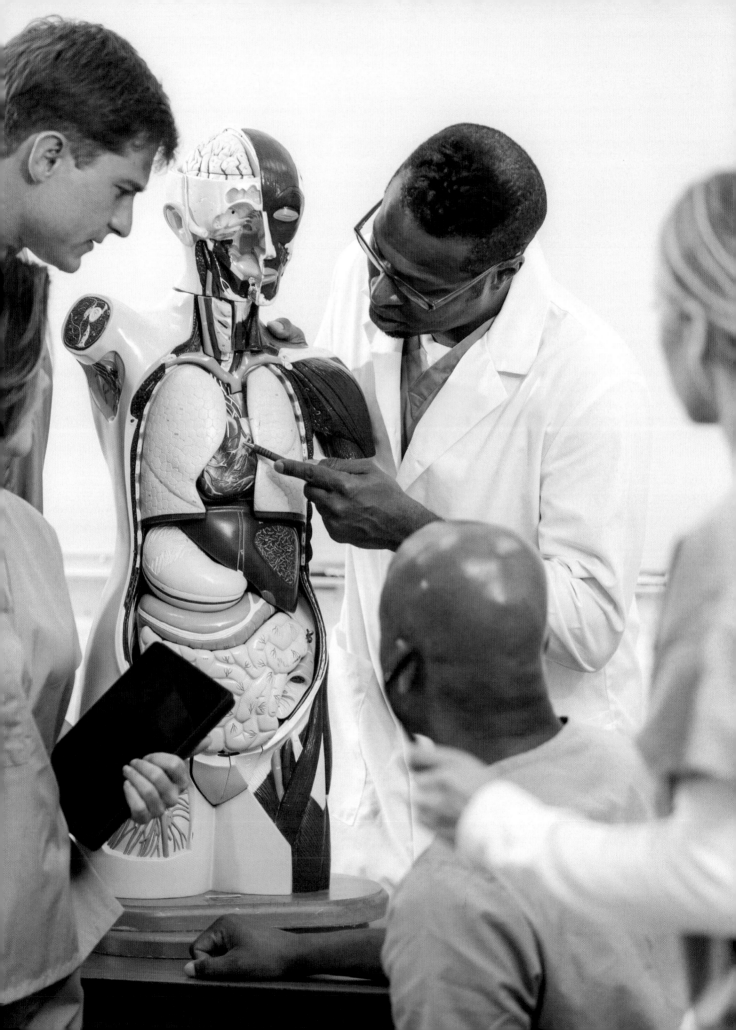

Assessment and feedback

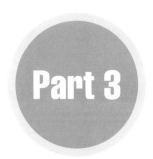

37 Feedback

Practice points

- Keeping the principles of giving effective feedback in mind helps both feedback giver and receiver
- Feedback is relational, it is part of a professional conversation and constructive dialogue
- Whilst feedback might occur 'in the moment', take time to plan and fully prepare when giving formal feedback

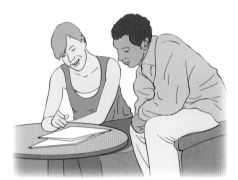

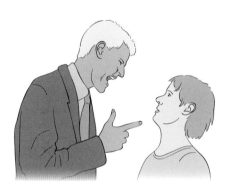

Box 37.1 Giving feedback

Do's

- Establish the learner's agenda
- Get the learner to start with what went well – the positive
- Teacher starts positive – however difficult it may seem
- Comment on specific aspects of the consultation – e.g. history taking – offer alternatives
- Active listening (eye contact, stance etc.), use silence
- Clarifying, responding to cues (verbal, non-verbal, psychosocial)
- Summarising, empathising etc.
- Move to areas "to be improved" (avoid the term "negative"!) – follow the learner's agenda first
- Begin with ".....I wonder if you had tried"
  "....perhaps you could have....."
  "...sometimes I find.....helpful...."
- Distinguish between the intention and the effect of a comment or behaviour
- Distinguish between the person and the performance ("what you said sounded judgmental" – rather than "You are judgmental")
- Do discuss clinical decision making
- Do be prepared to discuss ethical and attitudinal issues if they arise

Don'ts

- Don't forget the learner's emotional response – keep things safe
- Don't criticise without recommending improvements or different ways of doing things
- Don't comment on personal attributes that can't be changed
- Don't generalise – "you always" – but give specific examples
- Don't be dishonestly kind – if there is room for improvement be specific and explore alternative approaches
- Don't forget that your feedback says as much about you as about the person it is directed to!

Figure 37.1 Kolb's learning cycle

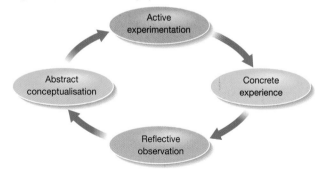

Figure 37.2 Johari window. Source: Luft and Ingham, 1955.

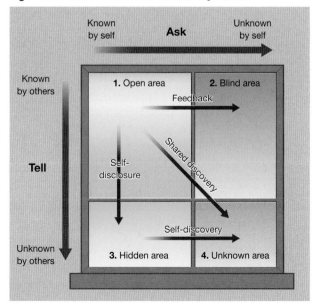

Whilst we all recognise that feedback is an essential part of all training and education programmes, however but all of us require ongoing feedback of some form or another – from an informal word of praise to a formal performance review/appraisal. Learners often say that they don't receive enough helpful feedback both on written work as well as in practice. It is important to set specific time aside for giving feedback (e.g. after an observed consultation or timetables into a medical programme after examination results) and flag up to learners that you are giving feedback. In an educational setting, feedback is not simply advice or praise, it is 'specific information about the comparison between… observed performance and a standard, given with the intent to improve… performance' (van der Ridder *et al.*, 2008). So what are the ways in which feedback can be delivered, how can we do it effectively and what do we do when it goes wrong?

Self-assessment alone is inadequate as the view of self that people have relates tenuously and modestly with the behaviour they exhibit and their performance (Dunning *et al.*, 2004). Accurate external feedback to learners is crucial, not only to enable them to consider the knowledge gap between actual and desired performance but to help them develop the capacity to critically evaluate their own (and others') performance and develop reflection. The **Johari window** (Figure 37.2) is a simple and effective model to increase self-awareness and encourage personal growth.

The Johari window invites people to *ask* for feedback about their performance and behaviours to learn more about themselves (decreases the *blind* pane) and to *tell* others about themselves so as to decrease the *hidden* pane. Effective feedback and professional conversations therefore encourages development of the *open* pane of the window.

Feedback and the learning process

It is important that feedback aligns with the overall learning outcomes of whatever activity in which the learner is engaged because reflecting on the activity encourages learning from that activity. Kolb (1984) proposed that learning is cyclical, that learning is experiential (learning by doing), and that ideas are formed and modified through experiences and reflection on those experiences (see Figure 37.1 and Chapter 5).

Principles of effective feedback

A number of models for giving effective feedback are available (e.g. Pendleton *et al.*, 1984; Silverman *et al.*, 1996; Walsh, 2005) but the main principles of feedback include those in Box 37.1 and the 'four Rs':

Relationship/rapport/respect: Good feedback needs to be set within the context of a good working relationship. It is a two-way dialogue between teacher and learner, with the teacher sharing knowledge and insights, and in return increasing their depth of understanding of their learner's needs.

Responsive/regular/routine: Feedback needs to be timely and regular and given in a manner sensitive to the learner's own perceptions. Care must be taken not to overload the learner, however, as too much feedback may have the opposite effect and decrease long term proficiency in learning (Schmidt, 1991).

Receptivity: Feedback needs to be constructive and therefore geared towards the learner's needs although closely aligned to the learning outcomes. Ideally, feedback should be 'feed forward', helping the learner to identify new goals, improvements or actions.

Rationalised: Feedback needs to be specifically focussed on observed behaviours rather than personality traits. It needs to be justified and non-judgemental. This means that when you are observing someone with a view to giving feedback, that you need to note down behaviours and dialogue so you can give specific examples such as 'when you were giving your Power-Point presentation, you turned to the screen at least five times and moved away from the microphone, so the participants couldn't hear what you were saying'.

Receiving feedback

Most teaching on feedback centres around delivery; however, the mechanisms by which feedback is received depend on the extent to which the recipient interprets, accepts and utilises the feedback they receive, that is the filter or the lens through which they receive the information. The degree to which feedback is deemed valuable by the learner is partly dependent on the extent with which the feedback resonates with their own self-assessment (Eva *et al.*, 2012). Feedback is more likely to be accepted and acted upon if it is learner directed, consistent and supportive. Guidelines for receiving constructive feedback include:

- Listening to it (rather than preparing your response/defence).
- Asking for it to be repeated if you did not hear it clearly.
- Assume it is constructive until proven otherwise; then consider and use those elements that are constructive.
- Pausing and thinking before responding.
- Asking for clarification and examples if statements are unclear or unsupported.
- Accepting it positively (for consideration) rather than dismissively (for self-protection).
- Asking for suggestions of ways you might modify or change your behavior.
- Respecting and thanking the person giving feedback.

Barriers to effective feedback

Fear of damaging the relationship from either teacher or learner may result in a reluctance to engage in the process, or to engage superficially. Feedback that is too generalised, non-specific or inconsistent (especially if coming from multiple sources) can result in feedback being negatively received. This can then have a detrimental effect on the person giving the feedback, which can further negatively impact the relationship (Hesketh and Laidlaw, 2002). Ultimately, feedback in education and healthcare settings should be based on a model of partnership. Treating learners as partners in their learning, just as we treat patients as partners in their health care is fundamental. The teacher is a partner with the learner and works alongside the learner whenever possible to achieve their desired outcomes. Just as some consultations 'go wrong', the same can be true for feedback conversations. It is important to use these as learning opportunities just like any other, to acknowledge the difficulties, identify the issues, reflect and move forward.

38 Principles of assessment

Figure 38.1 Assessment for the learner

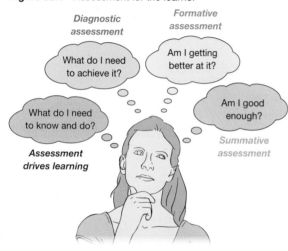

Figure 38.2 Assessment for institutions

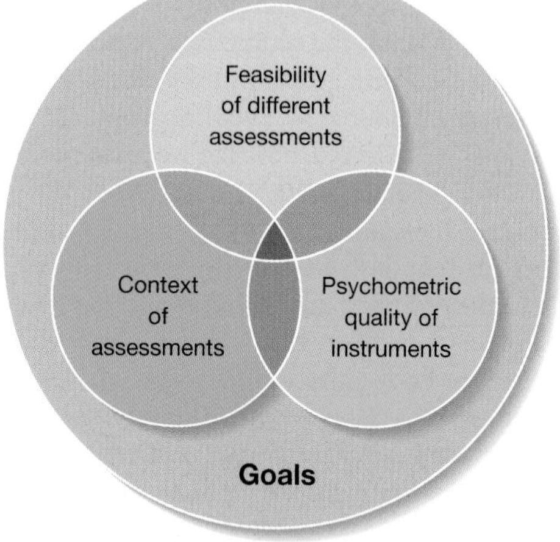

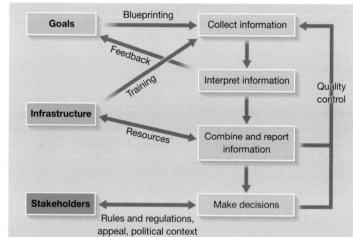

Figure 38.3 Elements involved in a programme of assessment

Figure 38.4 An example of a postgraduate programme of assessment

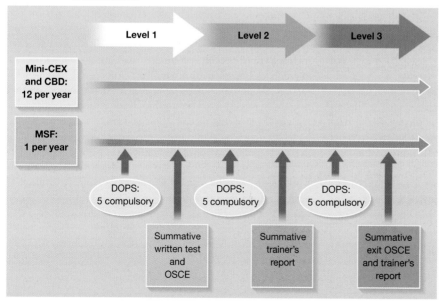

Abbrev: Mini-CEX, mini clinical evaluation exercise; CBD, case based discussion; MSF, multisource feedback; DOPS, direct observation of clinical skills; OSCE, objective structured clinical examination.

Medical Education at a Glance, First Edition. Edited by Judy McKimm, Kirsty Forrest and Jill Thistlethwaite © 2017 John Wiley & Sons, Ltd. Published 2017 by John Wiley & Sons, Ltd.

We assess learners to ensure they have met the defined learning outcomes or competencies required to move to the next level of education, training or practice. For certification or registration/preregistration as qualified medical practitioners, assessors must ensure that new doctors are fit to practise as interns (foundation year 1, or postgraduate year 1) and are safe. This is with the understanding that further learning and supervision are required for specialisation, and that doctors must be lifelong learners even without any further summative assessment.

The public expect that professionals should be assessed. The social contract between society and professionals assumes that doctors are qualified to practice and that they keep up to date. It is the responsibility of the appropriate accreditation body to set the standards for practice, and of medical schools and postgraduate bodies to develop curricula in accordance with these standards and to assess that learners meet them.

Assessment is also important for giving feedback to help learners improve (see Figure 38.1 and Chapter 37). The division of assessment into formative (assessment *for* learning) and summative (assessment *of* learning) is somewhat artificial: all assessment should be formative; however, this is not always the case. The term **diagnostic assessment** is applied to processes intended to explore learners' educational needs and help them develop learning plans. It is mainly used in postgraduate and continuing professional development (CPD).

Curriculum alignment

When planning assessments it is important to ensure that learning outcomes for a course or programme, and learning activities to meet those outcomes, are aligned across the curriculum (Biggs and Tang 2007). Learners need to know what they are expected to learn and what will be assessed. They also need to be aware that any learning outcome defined as part of the core curriculum could be assessed, therefore the common question 'is this going to be on the exam?' becomes irrelevant if learning activities are developed to meet core outcomes and are appropriate for the stage of training (see also Chapter 6).

Assessment blueprinting

Blueprinting is a technical component of assessment. It is the map that demonstrates curriculum alignment and shows where learning outcomes are being addressed, and when and how (e.g. through written tests such as multiple choice or short answer; clinically based, such as the objective structured clinical examination (OSCE); or work-based assessment) they are being assessed throughout a programme. Blueprinting is fundamental to test construction and item choice, ensuring that assessment is mapped carefully against learning outcomes to produce a valid examination (Dauphinée, 1994).

Definitions

There are at least seven attributes that should be considered when designing an assessment: validity, reliability, feasibility, cost effectiveness, educational impact, acceptability (van der Vleuten, 1996), and opportunity for feedback (Southgate and Grant, 2004). We would add to this authenticity, particularly in relation to clinical assessment (see also Figure 38.2).

Table 38.1 Definition of terms used in assessment

Term	Definition/explanation
Validity	How well an assessment measures what it is intended to measure; the degree to which the interpretation of scores resulting from an assessment activity are 'well grounded or justifiable' (Cook, 2014).
Predictive validity	How well an assessment is correlated with future observations of performance.
Reliability	The reproducibility of assessment scores between cohorts, over time and by different assessors. Inter-rater reliability (IRR) and agreement (IRA) assess the level of similarity between responses provided by different judges/observers.
Feasibility	Are there the resources including time, examiners/observers, patients, space and finance to carry out the assessment as developed? A cohort of 100 students for an OSCE, for example, is a very different proposition from a cohort of 300.
Acceptability	Assessments should be seen to be fair and equitable by all stakeholders. Students would consider it unacceptable to be examined on topics not covered in the curriculum.
Opportunity for feedback	An assessment is wasted in educational terms if learners do not learn from it. Consideration needs to be given to how learners may receive feedback on their performance, which should be timely, constructive and specific.
Educational impact	Assessments drive learning; assessments should be developed to stimulate learners to learn what is important and necessary. How may this impact be measured in the short and long term?
Cost effectiveness	Cost is not just financial but also includes time. Do the outcomes of an assessment merit the costs? Indeed, how are costs measured?
Authenticity	Assessment tasks are relevant and appropriate for the stage of learners and context; e.g. junior students should not be asked to play an intern in an OSCE, though this is acceptable for final year students.

High stakes assessments should be valid and reliable. This increases their acceptability to stakeholders including those assessing and those being assessed. Assessments need to be seen as fair and trustworthy. Double marking may increase acceptability, particularly for clinical examinations such as the OSCE, but may not be feasible. Many medical schools have large student cohorts, some over 300. Finding the resources (space, assessors, time) for such large numbers can be difficult and costly if simulated patients and assessors are paid.

The assessors

Traditionally assessors/examiners have been senior doctors or educators – experts in the field. More recently, peer and near-peer assessment has become more widespread particularly for group and team-based activities, and work-based assessment. The role of patients in assessment is an important consideration, with a move from passive to active involvement (see Chapter 21).

Programmatic assessment

Learning and assessment should occur in cycles, with aggregated assessment data points longitudinally throughout a programme, rather than one-off single assessments (Figures 38.3 and 38.4). Individual data points are then maximised for learning and feedback value, and summative decisions are based on the aggregation of many points. Fundamental to this process is sampling across a range of assessment types and contexts, thus reducing bias because of the inherent subjectivity of examiner judgements (van der Vleuten *et al.*, 2012).

39 Written assessments

Practice points

- Written assessments should form part of an overall assessment strategy
- Institutions are now frequently sharing their banks of questions in return for new items for the bank
- Machine markable assessments take time to write but are quick to mark and provide psychometric data

Table 39.1 Strengths and weaknesses of some different types of written question format

Question type	Marking	Response format	Advantages	Disadvantages
Single best answer (SBA) /best of five/ multiple choice question (MCQ)	Machine markable	Closed	Flexible Easy to administer Cover a broad range of topics in a short time Give reliable scores per hour of testing time Test application of knowledge Test a range of areas, e.g. assessment, investigation, treatment	Can have redundant distracters Can cue the right answer Need practice to write well Difficult to test higher-order skills
Multiple true false (MTF)	Machine markable	Closed	Easy to administer Cover a broad range of topics in a short time Test a range of areas	Only test factual recall Can be easy to guess
Extended matching question (EMQ)	Machine markable	Closed	Focus on problem solving May reduce cueing	Less coverage of topics Hard to find homogenous options for all vignettes Better for diagnosis than other elements
Short answer question	Human markers	Open-ended	Can test in 'grey' areas	Take longer to answer Less coverage of topics Need expert markers Need a clearly defined answer key Can lack clarity
Essay question / modified essay question (MEQ)	Human markers	Open-ended	Can test reasoning and application of complex concepts, including 'grey' areas Can test analytical skills	Take longer to answer Less coverage of topics Need expert markers Need a clearly defined answer key In MEQs, if get first part wrong will likely get all parts wrong

Figure 39.1 Example of a single best answer (SBA) question

Stem: A 5-year-old girl has had a headache most days for the last 4 weeks. It is worse in the mornings and eased by paracetamol. She was still going to school but for the last week she has been vomiting on waking up every day and says her 'tummy' hurts.

Lead-in: Which is the single most likely diagnosis?

Options:
A. Abdominal migraine
B. Brain tumour
C. Epstein Barr virus infection
D. Idiopathic intracranial hypertension
E. Tension headache

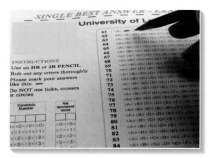

Figure 39.2 Item analysis data following a computer marked test

Item analysis report

Exam statistics: mean 85.2 (72.6%), st.dev: 16.1 (13.79%), candidates: 224, KR20: 0.89

Question 61

		Thirds	Right	Wrong	R-W	Void
Mean score	1.464	% all	73.2	26.8	46.4	0.0
33% item discrimination	0.439	Upper	94.7	5.3	89.5	0.0
Point biserial	0.342	Lower	50.9	49.1	1.8	0.0
Correct answer	B	Facility	73.2			

% Answer frequency

Multi	Blank	A	B	C	D	E
0.0	0.0	17.9	73.2	0.0	5.4	3.6

Medical Education at a Glance, First Edition. Edited by Judy McKimm, Kirsty Forrest and Jill Thistlethwaite © 2017 John Wiley & Sons, Ltd. Published 2017 by John Wiley & Sons, Ltd.

Written assessments are used in a variety of medical settings across the world, from undergraduate end-of-year exams to postgraduate licensing and specialist qualifications. Part of the reason they remain popular is their ease of administration. They allow reliable and standardised testing for large numbers of candidates at a relatively low cost. However, they should be only one part of an overall assessment strategy to test clinical competence. Written assessments generally achieve testing at the bottom two levels of Miller's Pyramid; 'knows' and 'knows how' (Miller, 1990).

Types of written question

A number of different formats can be used, each of which has advantages and disadvantages (Table 39.1). Not all question types are mentioned here, although the main ones in use are. They can be broadly categorised in two ways:

1 Machine markable versus human marked
2 Closed question format versus open-ended format.

Clearly, machine-markable tests are easier to administer to large cohorts. The commonest question type in use in UK assessments is the SBA (single best answer), sometimes known as a best of five or an MCQ. While some argue that these questions are not suited to testing higher order cognitive skills, evidence shows that the response format itself is not as important as the stimulus, that is what you ask and how you ask it. An example of an SBA is shown in Figure 39.1. This type of SBA does not simply test knowledge recall, such as what is the incubation period for hepatitis A, but if written as a clinical scenario requires application of knowledge. EMQs (extended matching questions) are written around a theme, such as causes of headache, and a long list of options is presented followed by a number of clinical vignettes. The candidate selects one correct option from the list for each vignette. MTF (multiple true false) questions allow candidates to select either true or false for a number of statements around an issue or case.

While many medical schools still use open-ended format questions, these are notoriously difficult to standardise and require much more time and resource in the form of human markers. They are, therefore, less popular. Short-answer questions ask a candidate to write a few words in answer to a specific question. Essay questions require longer answers, although they can be broken down into specific subheadings in MEQs (modified essay questions), which may follow a patient case from diagnosis to management for example. Other forms of assessment, such as the OSCE (objective structured clinical examination), may also be used to assess higher order skills, such as clinical reasoning, as part of an overall assessment strategy (see Chapter 40).

The key message is that there is no *right* type of question. Different question formats will suit different purposes. It is important to be clear about what it is you are trying to test, to understand the advantages and disadvantages of different methods, and to decide where your written assessment fits into an overall assessment of clinical competence using a variety of instruments.

Tips for writing good questions

Writing good test questions is far from straightforward. Published guides are available that go into detail on specific question types. Generally, though, questions are best written in small groups, with consultation before they are used live. Groups should include content experts as well as well-experienced question writers. Sentences should always be clear, concise and use plain language while containing all necessary information. A reviewer can check that a question actually asks what was intended. In SBAs, a good candidate should ideally be able to give the answer without seeing the options – the cover test. The question should be set at the right level for the learners being assessed and be congruent with the appropriate learning outcomes for the stage of learning.

It is obviously important that the correct answer is actually correct and that incorrect ones are definitely incorrect. This can be trickier than it sounds and is another reason why review is so helpful, for both closed-format questions and in constructing the answer key for open-ended questions. In closed formats, answers should all be homogenous, logical and ideally all the same sort of length to prevent candidates easily choosing one over the other. It is usually fairly straightforward to find three plausible options for an SBA, but finding four or five can be more difficult. However, despite evidence showing that candidates rarely actually choose between more than three options, five remains the standard number. It is equally tricky finding an homogenous set of eight or more options for an EMQ. Therefore, they risk simply becoming a set of SBAs, all on the same theme.

Quality control

The quality of an assessment depends on the quality of individual items so it is vital to do as much quality control as possible *before* using items in testing situations, particularly in high-stakes summative assessments. This means review by both content and assessment experts, blueprinting items to the curriculum (see Chapter 38) and, occasionally, trialling items beforehand. A great deal of data can be gathered when an item is used in a testing situation and much of this can be helpful for item design and feedback.

When machine-markable tests are marked, the software package will generally give you psychometric data about the whole test and each item. While it will depend on the cohort tested, these data can be helpful in spotting item flaws. A good item will discriminate between competent students, who do well overall, and those who have not achieved competence. It will also be relevant to the curriculum and not too hard or too easy. Figure 39.2 shows an example of data generated about an SBA question.

If you have the luxury of a large bank of questions and enthusiastic writers, you may be able to test items in situ during an assessment, with such items not being included in the final mark.

Written assessments are therefore good for testing knowledge and application of knowledge and can be delivered to large cohorts feasibly, reliably and at relatively low cost. However, good-quality control procedures are needed to ensure that the right types of question are used depending on the testing situation, and that individual items are constructed to the highest quality.

40 # Assessment of clinical skills

Practice points

- Clinical skills assessments test either competence (what a learner or practitioner is able to do) or performance (what they actually do in practice)
- The Objective Structured Clinical Examination (OSCE) is the most commonly used assessment of clinical competence
- Whilst OSCEs are resource intensive, they have high levels of reliability and validity

Figure 40.1   Schematic of an OSCE circuit

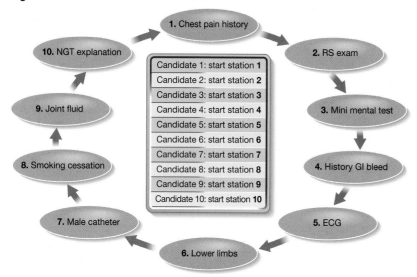

1. Chest pain history
2. RS exam
3. Mini mental test
4. History GI bleed
5. ECG
6. Lower limbs
7. Male catheter
8. Smoking cessation
9. Joint fluid
10. NGT explanation

Candidate 1: start station **1**
Candidate 2: start station **2**
Candidate 3: start station **3**
Candidate 4: start station **4**
Candidate 5: start station **5**
Candidate 6: start station **6**
Candidate 7: start station **7**
Candidate 8: start station **8**
Candidate 9: start station **9**
Candidate 10: start station **10**

Table 40.1   Example of an OSCE blueprint

	Information gathering – history	Information gathering – examination	Practical technical skills	Information giving	Data analysis
Cardiovascular	Chest pain history		ECG performance and interpretation ———————————————→		
Respiratory		RS exam		Smoking cessation advice	
GI / GU	History GI bleed		Male catheter ———————————————→		

Figure 40.2   Example of a checklist-based OSCE mark sheet

University Medical School
Final year OSCE
Examiner Marksheet
Station 2

A = outstanding B = good C = adequate D = marginal E = inadequate

1. Introduces self to patient
2. Positions patient at 45°
3. Examines surroundings
4. Examines periphery from hands to neck
5. Exposes and inspects chest wall fully
6. Palpates trachea and apex beat
7. Checks for expansion front and back
8. Percusses in 6 areas front and back
9. Auscultates in 6 area front and back
10. Checks vocal fremitus in 6 areas front and back
11. Correctly interprets findings

A B C D E

Global Rating	6	5	4	3	2	1
	EXCELLENT	VERY GOOD	CLEAR PASS	BORDERLINE PASS	BORDERLINE FAIL	CLEAR FAIL

Please mark in the box as shown, using the pencil provided

Figure 40.3   Example of a domain-based OSCE mark sheet

University Medical School
Final year OSCE
Examiner Marksheet
Station 1

A = outstanding B = good C = adequate D = marginal E = inadequate

1. Initial approach to patient
2. Information gathering/history: clinical content
3. Information gathering/history: communication skills
4. Rapport and professionalism
5. SP mark

A B C D E

Global Rating	6	5	4	3	2	1
	EXCELLENT	VERY GOOD	CLEAR PASS	BORDERLINE PASS	BORDERLINE FAIL	CLEAR FAIL

Please mark in the box as shown, using the pencil provided

Medical Education at a Glance, First Edition. Edited by Judy McKimm, Kirsty Forrest and Jill Thistlethwaite © 2017 John Wiley & Sons, Ltd. Published 2017 by John Wiley & Sons, Ltd.

A clinical practitioner uses a variety of skills in the workplace. Assessing these is clearly far more complex than testing knowledge using a pen and paper. Over the last 30 years a number of assessments of clinical skills have been developed and validated. These either test clinical competence – what a student or practitioner is *able to do* – or performance – what they *actually do* in practice. Performance assessments take place in the workplace (see Chapter 41). Tests of clinical competence take place in artificial settings and have the advantage of being able to assess many individuals at the same time in a standardised way.

The Objective Structured Clinical Examination

The Objective Structured Clinical Examination (OSCE), introduced in the 1970s (Harden *et al.*, 1975), is the most widely used assessment of clinical skills. It comprises a series of structured, timed stations around which each candidate moves in sequence. Each station tests a particular clinical skill, or set of skills, and involves varying degrees of simulation: manikins, part task trainers, simulated patients (SPs), computer-based simulation or a combination of these. Sometimes 'real' or standardised patients are used with specific signs. Each candidate completes the same set of tasks in the same time, moving around a circuit (Figure 40.1). The length of each station needs to be just long enough for a competent candidate to complete the task. Stations are usually the same length in a circuit although sometimes double stations are used for more complex tasks. Each station is marked by a different examiner, who completes a structured score sheet that has been determined in advance. The OSCE is typically used in summative assessments, at both undergraduate and postgraduate level. It has been shown to have high levels of reliability and validity due to having high numbers of stations marked independently in a structured way.

Organising an OSCE

While they play a central role in the assessment of clinical skills, OSCEs can be time consuming and difficult to organise. Planning needs to begin, ideally, several months in advance and a dedicated team of people is needed to run a large OSCE well. Top tips for running a successful OSCE are:

- Have a standard operating procedure detailing what will be done, when and by whom.
- Draw up a blueprint well in advance (Table 40.1) that is mapped to the curriculum; give people deadlines to write each station.
- Carefully calculate how many candidates you have, how many stations you need, how long each complete circuit will be, how many circuits you can run alongside one another and how many sessions you will need.
- Start recruiting examiners to fill all stations, circuits and sessions well before the exam, and always recruit a couple of extras.
- Ensure all examiners are trained and know what their roles are.
- Compile a list of resources needed – actors, volunteers, manikins, equipment – and assign someone to arrange these.

- Pilot all new stations to make sure they work as expected.
- Expect the unexpected on the day of the OSCE itself. Make sure there are plenty of people on the ground to troubleshoot.

Writing an OSCE station

A good station will be based on a real clinical encounter, have a clear construct, test specific clinical skills, be achievable in the time allowed and minimise potential sources of bias or error. This is hard to get right, and review by peers and experts and trial runs are vital to anticipate all potential problems. Remember:

- Don't try to cram too much in to the station.
- Think carefully about the task you are asking the candidates to do and make the instructions clear and specific.
- Make instructions for actors/SPs clear, comprehensive and realistic – consider all possible avenues the candidate might take.
- Consider what elements should be scored and what the candidate will gain marks for, bearing in mind their teaching.
- Make the examiner's part as small as possible – don't build in viva questions.

Scoring OSCEs

The two main types of scoring are checklist based and domain based (Figures 40.2 and 40.3). Checklist style mark sheets are more suited to novice practitioners who are just learning a skill and practise it in a fairly rigid way (Boursicot *et al.*, 2011). Domain-based scoring systems award marks in domains of practice, such as approach to the patient or information gathering, and allow more flexibility. They are usually coupled with anchor statements, or guides for examiners on what is expected to gain marks. Whichever system is used, marks can be weighted to attach more importance to certain aspects of the skill. Generally, examiners are also asked to give a *global* overall rating of performance to aid standard setting (see Chapter 44). Assessors are used, although the patient (real or simulated) may be asked to award a judgement in an agreed domain, such as communication.

OSCEs and the hidden curriculum?

When designing an OSCE, thought has to be given to the unspoken messages educators are giving learners. For example, having 7-minute stations for breaking bad news suggests that certain complex tasks can be done well in such a short time in clinical practice.

Other types of clinical skills' assessment

The OSCE replaced the traditional long case, which was inherently variable and unreliable. However, the Objective Structured Long Case Examination Record (OSLER) involves standardised patients and structured mark schemes to allow assessment of a whole patient encounter rather than a part task; large numbers are needed for reliability (Gleeson, 1997). Various surgical specialities have also developed their own variations on the OSCE to assess specific surgical skills.

41 Work-based assessment

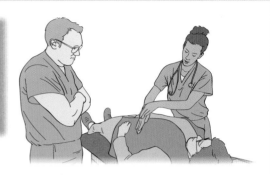

Practice points

- Work-based assessment (WBA) focuses on assessment of performance in everyday clinical practice
- Many different types of WBA are now being used
- WBA has problems with reliability but, over time, is useful for formative assessment to support learning
- Multiple assessments by different people over time helps improve the reliability of WBA for individual learners

Table 41.1 Multi-source feedback form: example of some typical questions

To be filled in by colleagues, peers, supervisors, members of other health professions as appropriate

How do you rate this medical student/doctor in relation to their:	Good	Satisfactory	Needs to improve	Unacceptable	Unable to comment
Clinical knowledge					
Clinical skills					
Communication with patients					
Communication with families					
Communication with colleagues					
Teamwork					
Awareness of own limitations					
Readiness to seek help appropriately					
Ability to time manage and prioritise					
Record keeping					
Showing respect					
Maintaining confidentiality					
Treating others without bias or discrimination					
Cultural awareness					
Honesty and integrity					
Taking responsibility for their actions					
I would recommend them to a friend or family member	Yes	No			

Figure 41.1 Examples of a mini-clinical exercise (mini-CEX) form

Source: *Understanding Medical Education: Evidence, Theory and Practice*, 2nd edn. Edited by Tim Swanwick. © 2014 The Association for the Study of Medical Education. Published 2014 by John Wiley & Sons, Ltd. Reproduced with permission of John Wiley & Sons.

Work-based assessment (WBA) focuses on assessment of performance in everyday clinical practice, rather than of competence under controlled conditions such as in the Objective Structured Clinical Examination (OSCE) (Chapter 40). WBA assesses at the 'does' level of Miller's pyramid (Miller, 1990). Even in the workplace, in clinical environments, a single demonstration of competence at one time (for example an assessment of one consultation) is not enough to prove adequate performance in the workplace, from day to day. The gap between competence and performance was identified several decades ago (Rethans *et al.*, 1991) with subsequent recognition of the importance of work-based assessment to bridge this gap. Performance is the ability to do the job well, what doctors do in their professional practice (Rethans *et al.*, 2002) and is assessed 'on the job' in clinical practice. WBA is also referred to as workplace-based assessment.

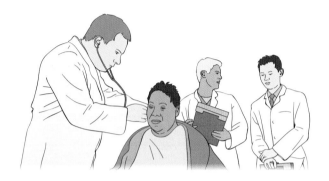

Types of WBA

A growing number of methods of assessment are used pre- and postqualification of which the first three below are most commonly used:
- Mini-clinical exercise (mini-CEX).
- Directly observed assessment of practical skills (DOPS).
- Case-based discussions (CBDs) of patients the learner has managed with a more senior clinician; explores understanding of particular cases focussing on the whole case or a particular aspect.
- Shift report during which a trainee is observed for the duration of a clinical shift.
- 360-degree evaluation (multisource feedback, MSF) – structured feedback is gathered from a range of sources including from nurses and other health professionals, receptionists, senior and junior colleagues, and sometimes patients. Respondents may be invited by a supervisor or the individual requiring feedback (Table 41.1). Data are anonymised and may not be timely or constructive.
- Incognito/unannounced simulated/standardised patients in consultations – not commonly used except in the Netherlands as the method has numerous logistical, and some feel ethical, issues.
- Videotaped consultations in clinical settings with real (not simulated) patients.
- Patient satisfaction surveys – tend to focus on communication and professionalism; these are anonymised to ensure patient care is not compromised in future.
- Patient quality of care and outcome data through audits and computerised records – not commonly used during training but often linked to payment in some countries.

Requirements for the number and timing of WBA at the various levels of education and training vary across jurisdictions and specialties.

Rationale

WBA should provide a framework for supporting and improving learning and teaching. As such, it falls under the heading of assessment *for* learning and is an opportunity for structured feedback and discussion between observer and observed. However, WBA instruments have also been developed to improve the validity and the authenticity of judgments of performance. A series of WBA may be used in conjunction with other in-training assessments (ITA) to provide evidence that a doctor in training or student is fit to progress to the next level of training, or requires remediation.

To improve reliability and objectivity, complex and context-specific clinical tasks have been broken down into discrete elements in some WBA. For example, during the mini-CEX a learner (student or doctor in training) interacts with a patient to elicit a history and carry out a physical examination (Norcini *et al.*, 2003) and is rated on interviewing, examination and counselling skills, professionalism and communication, clinical judgement and organisation/efficiency (Figure 41.1). However, even with the most detailed grade descriptors for each of these skills or tasks, there is an element of personal opinion (Kogan *et al.*, 2009), which is acknowledged by the common addition of a **global rating** independent of the accrued grades on the checklist. While the focus is on observation and feedback by a sole assessor the fact that the inter-rater reliability of the mini-CEX is variable may not be a major issue. Formal assessor training has not shown a consistent effect on improving the reliability of rating (Boursicot *et al.*, 2011).

Evaluation

A systematic review of WBA from 2010 looked at the published evidence as to its impact on doctors' learning and performance (Miller and Archer, 2010). It found that while many papers describe WBA, its development and implementation, few consider educational impact. The authors conclude that there is only objective evidence that MSF can lead to improvement, though subjective data from doctors in training and assessors suggest that the mini-CEX, DOPS and CBDs did improve the quality of training. The feedback process in MSF is certainly important, as is the impact of negative feedback.

Difficulties

While the mini-CEX does mimic the task of a medical student or doctor in training, checklists of discrete elements are 'at least in part, responsible for what might be described variously as "reductionist", "deconstructive", "tick-box", "mechanistic" or "instrumentalist' approaches to assessment' and 'the lack of appreciation of assessment as the learning tool for the student' (Amin, 2012, p. 5). Without a feedback dialogue, WBA can become just something to 'get through' during training. In busy clinical settings it may be difficult for learners to find an appropriate clinician to observe them, who also has the time for the feedback process. In addition, although patients are involved in the mini-CEX, they are not necessarily asked for their opinion on the learner's or professional's performance. Patient feedback may be gathered as part of the MSF or through separate patient satisfaction questionnaire but this does not allow discussion, unlike learning through a simulated patient activity.

42 Assessing professionalism

Practice points

- Assessing professionalism is a very complex and evolving field
- Academic assessment of professional behaviours should be carried out using multiple assessment tools and assessors, and must include work-based assessment
- Unprofessional behaviour may lead to fitness to practise procedures, but these must be clearly distinguished from the academic assessment process

Figure 42.1 Example of professional assessment blueprinting

Assessment modality	Summative								Formative	
	MSF	OSCE	MiniCEX	Clinical placement	SSCs/cases	Simulation	Reflection	Patient feedback	Concern forms	Academic record
Personal qualities										
Demonstrates honesty/integrity	✓	✓	✓	✓			✓	✓		
Punctual/good timekeeping and attendance	✓	✓	✓	✓		✓				
Respects others views/opinions	✓					✓	✓	✓		
Appropriate dress		✓	✓	✓		✓				
Reliable	✓		✓	✓		✓				
Insightful/thoughtful/reflective						✓	✓		✓	
Knows own limits and boundaries	✓			✓		✓	✓			
Handles emotions appropriately	✓	✓	✓			✓	✓	✓		
Listens	✓	✓	✓	✓		✓		✓		
Copes well under pressure		✓		✓		✓				
Working with colleagues										
Works constructively in the team	✓			✓	✓	✓	✓			
Understands/maintains professional boundaries	✓		✓	✓	✓	✓	✓			
Understands impact of behaviour on others	✓			✓	✓	✓	✓			
Shows appropriate leadership					✓	✓				
Working with patients		✓	✓	✓				✓		
Supportive/helped my learning	✓			✓				✓		
Working with patients										
Demonstrates caring/empathy/compassion	✓	✓	✓	✓	✓		✓	✓		
Advocates for patients/families		✓	✓	✓			✓			
Communicates appropriately		✓	✓	✓	✓		✓	✓		
Gives understandable information		✓	✓	✓		✓	✓	✓		
Demonstrates ethical approach		✓	✓	✓			✓	✓		
Understands limits of own role/abilities		✓	✓	✓	✓	✓	✓	✓		
Working with tasks										
Understands and applies the law		✓	✓	✓	✓	✓	✓			
Engages with activities well			✓	✓	✓	✓	✓			
Prioritises appropriately and meets deadlines			✓	✓			✓			✓

(Assessable behaviours)

Figure 42.2 Example (part only) of end of clinical placement assessment form

Part 2: Professionalism and values

Scope of practice – This student (please tick one option that applies):
- Sought opportunities to extend their expertise within safe boundaries
- Practised safely whilst recognising their own limitations
- Struggled to recognise own strengths and weaknesses and required advice to take full advantage of the learning opportunities available
- Practised unsafely and failed to understand their own boundaries and/or the limitations of their role[1,2]

Communicating with all colleagues – This student (please tick one option that applies):
- Consistently demonstrated excellent communication skills, whenever observed
- Communicated effectively and appropriately at all times, when observed
- Initially required guidance on effective and appropriate communication and has now improved to the required standard
- Demonstrated significant deficiencies in communication skills despite guidance

Patient advocacy – This student (please tick one option that applies):
- Consistently demonstrated caring, compassionate, respectful, advocatory patient centred care
- Initially failed to demonstrate patient centred care but improved with guidance
- Consistently failed to demonstrate patient centred care

1 Examples of unprofessional behaviour include: inappropriate dress, dishonesty, lack of respect, failure to demonstrate an ethical approach to practice, failure to understand legal principles in practice, difficulties handling their emotions, lack of insight and reflection.
2 A serious lapse in professional behaviour should also prompt completion of a student concern form.

With acknowledgments to Swansea University

Medical Education at a Glance, First Edition. Edited by Judy McKimm, Kirsty Forrest and Jill Thistlethwaite © 2017 John Wiley & Sons, Ltd. Published 2017 by John Wiley & Sons, Ltd.

The complexity of defining the attributes, competencies and behaviours that comprise 'professionalism' in practice means that assessments need to consider: knowledge and understanding; practical skills and procedures; problem-solving abilities; and behaviours that reflect attitudes and characteristics. Behaviours must be assessed in context as learners may act unprofessionally when they feel pressured to do so, for example examining a very unwell patient just because they have 'good signs'. Alternatively, they may 'fake' professional behaviours when they feel they are being observed and behave differently when working independently.

Assessing professionalism is one of the most challenging areas to assess and Goldie's (2013) review summarises the approach to assessing professionalism as an evolving field. Because it is a multidimensional construct, dependent on cultural contexts, individuals, teams and situations, then a longitudinal, multidimensional approach needs to be taken. Assessments need to be both *for learning* (developmental) and *of learning* (checking knowledge or practical competence). Increasingly, professionalism assessment is mapped into domains (e.g. working with other professionals or punctuality), which are tested longitudinally and blueprinted across a range of assessments (see Figure 42.1 for an example). This approach can help highlight areas of particular strength or in need of improvement.

Formal assessment might sometimes give rise to a professional concerns or incident report for individual learners (e.g. being rude to a 'patient' in an OSCE) and may highlight support needs or fitness to practise issues. Care must be taken however to clearly separate assessment of academic professional behaviours or understanding from fitness to practice processes, although similar issues (e.g. persistent lateness or plagiarism) may arise and be considered through both processes.

As with any assessment, the methods chosen need to be reliable, valid, feasible and acceptable (see Chapter 38 for definitions).

Written assessment

Paper assessments or computer based tests can be useful when assessing the knowledge or understanding which underpins professional practice (see Chapter 39). Typical assessments include:

Case studies with patients/families: these can be designed to assess understanding of professional issues (such as ethical issues) in depth, including an empathic understanding of the patient's perspective and reflective narratives.

Service or quality improvement projects (including audits), which assess understanding of health service changes, evidence based practice and the role of the learner as a change champion.

Multiple choice questions (MCQs): these are useful for checking knowledge of specific issues (e.g. the law, professional bodies' requirements) as well as applying knowledge to practice, for example through clinical vignettes.

Situational judgement tests (SJTs) are currently used more in selection (see Chapter 9). Learners have to rank their responses to professional dilemma-based scenarios. There is not usually one clear answer, but some are better (or worse) than others.

Significant event or critical incident analyses can be used to assess learner's analysis (understanding) and reflections on and for action regarding a positive or negative event of significance to them.

Portfolios are useful for assessing reflection, insight and understanding of the impact of actions on others (see Chapter 43).

Practical assessment

Practical assessments, whether of single competencies (e.g. inserting a nasogastric tube, taking blood) or assessing multiple, complex high-level competencies (e.g. managing emergency situations) can be undertaken under test conditions or in the workplace. Whilst assessment of professionalism does not specifically consider technical skills or procedures, it is difficult to disentangle these, particularly in the workplace. The most common instrument used is the OSCE (Objective Structured Clinical Examination) which includes a number of stations testing different competencies of varying levels of complexity (see Chapter 40). The OSCE is designed to test a combination of practical skills, written ability and verbal and non-verbal behaviours. Stations that test professional behaviours and understanding may include video or computer-based ethical scenarios as well as clinical and communication skills' assessments (e.g. showing respect or empathy or giving information appropriately) using simulators, manikins, actors, simulated patients or real patients.

Work-based assessment

These are generally considered to be the most valid tests of professional practice when carried out on multiple occasions, by different assessors, in different contexts (see Chapter 41). Most programmes include an end of placement assessment of learners' performance completed by the supervising clinician and/or their team. This is usually a checklist which asks various questions relating to clinical abilities as well as how the learner worked with the team, with patients and families, their timekeeping, etc. (see Figure 42.2).

One issue found in practice is that clinicians are often unwilling to 'fail' learners and may not report 'minor' unprofessional behaviours as they may think this could lead to sanction (Ypres-Roi *et al.*, 2015). However, repeated occurrences of such 'low level' behaviours can indicate a need for remediation or a fitness to practise issue, so encouraging open recording of these behaviours is important.

Some work-based assessments are more global, for example the P-MEX (professional mini-evaluation exercise) considers four sets of professional skills. Other instruments (e.g. the Mini-CEX) focus on specific aspects of clinical performance or observed clinical encounters and incorporate professional domains within them.

Feedback

Ideally, all assessments of professionalism should aim to encourage and facilitate learning and reflection. Feedback is an important part of learning. Feedback needs to be timely, focussed on improving performance or highlighting unhelpful behaviours, use specific examples and be constructive. Multisource (or 360 degree) feedback (MSF) is a specific approach that aims to gather and collate standardised feedback from a number of peers, colleagues or patients in a systematic way. MSF is a powerful tool for development if used well but feedback needs to be given carefully and with support, especially if negative. Patient surveys are becoming increasingly common for practising clinicians. Chapter 37 looks more closely at the role of feedback in developing reflective practice.

Self-rating

Many examples of self-rating forms exist relating to professionalism; some are free online resources, others have to be administered through an organisation. These include scales on empathy, resilience, time management, reflection, cultural competency, team working, leadership and personality preferences. If used with care, they can help learners develop self-insight and understanding.

43 Portfolios

Box 43.1 Portfolio contents

Possible medical student contents

- Tutor reports
- Evidence of communication skills
- Skills log with evidence of attainment
- Evidence of meeting professionalism outcomes
- Certificates or awards
- Assessment results
- Reflective diary

Postgraduate/revalidation contents

- Learning plans
- Certificates of attendance at courses
- Work-based assessment forms
- Critical incident analysis/significant event audit
- Clinical audit activity
- Patient satisfaction forms
- Peer review of teaching

Figure 43.1 Assessing using portfolios

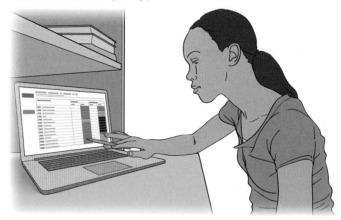

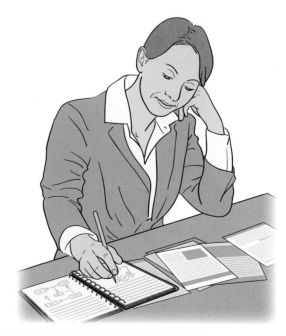

Medical Education at a Glance, First Edition. Edited by Judy McKimm, Kirsty Forrest and Jill Thistlethwaite © 2017 John Wiley & Sons, Ltd. Published 2017 by John Wiley & Sons, Ltd.

Portfolios are purposeful collections of work to demonstrate a person's ability within a particular field. The word originally referred to the object containing the work that allowed it to be portable. The contents are evidence of something: for example drawings and paintings are evidence of an artist's ability. In medical education, portfolios are a collection of documents (or other materials such as audiotapes, videos) that help provide evidence that learning has taken place, as well as some form of reflection on documented events (Snadden and Thomas, 1998).

Portfolios are frequently required to show that learners have reached the required standard for their level of training. For doctors this includes evidence of fitness to practise and appropriate professional attributes. In the UK, the 5-yearly revalidation cycle requires doctors to keep a portfolio that is discussed at their annual appraisals. Professional medical educators also need to develop a portfolio, which may include evidence of teaching and learning, evaluations and qualifications in education.

The contents depend on the purpose of the portfolio and its role in formative and summative assessment. They may be very strictly defined and structured, or more flexible and learner centred.

The rationale for portfolio-based assessment

In many countries, doctors need to provide evidence of continuing professional development (CPD) in order to continue to be licensed or registered to practise. Revalidation of doctors in the UK is a formal example of this process. Medical schools, by ensuring that students are familiar with maintaining a portfolio as a record of their learning and competence, ease them into the habit of collecting evidence from an early stage of their careers. In addition, portfolios are useful tools for demonstrating professional development.

Personal and professional development (PPD) courses and professionalism outcomes focus on communication and interpersonal skills, ethics and values, self-care, critical analysis and working in teams. Evidence of achieving outcomes or competencies in these areas at the appropriate standard can be ideal material for inclusion in portfolios.

Personal development plans

At a basic level a portfolio is a learning plan with evidence.

Learning plan: A list of learning outcomes or competencies to be achieved.

Personal development plan (PDP): Educational priorities for a set period of time. Should include how the priorities are identified, how learning is to be achieved and what evidence will be collected to show achievement.

The crucial elements of a PDP include what needs to be learned, how you know you need to learn it and (to close the loop) how you know you have learned it. As the name implies, PDPs should be personal and should therefore be unique to an individual. However, students need guidance, especially in their early years. Learning outcomes are defined in the formal curriculum but students still need to be able to reflect on whether these have been met.

Trigger questions, including PUNs and DENs (patient's unmet needs, doctor's educational needs) in clinical practice (Eve, 2003), are helpful for setting personal outcomes across the continuum of education.

What do portfolios look like?

An institution, profession or specialty may stipulate what a portfolio should look like, particularly if it is to be used for summative assessment; uniformity helps assessors find their way around the contents. Paper-based portfolios can be difficult to carry around. Care needs to be taken about confidentiality and anonymity of contents – any data relating to patients should not be identifiable.

E-portfolios

Evidence may be collected and stored electronically. E-portfolios are portable and accessible at multiple locations if cloud based. However there may also be issues of confidentiality and access should be protected.

Assessment of portfolios

Given the large number of medical students at some schools, the assessment of portfolios represents a tremendous undertaking in terms of resources. For summative assessment there are issues of reliability (how many assessors are required?). For formative assessment, portfolios need to be reviewed to check progress and responses to feedback. Ideally, some form of appraisal or interview process should be undertaken with each learner so that feedback becomes a dialogue and the process itself becomes part of the evidence. Certainly students who produce below standard portfolios should have a chance to discuss their work with a tutor/faculty member. Of course this raises the question of how the standard is set, and whether there is a pass mark or grading system.

Driessen *et al.* (2005) have advised that the interpretation of portfolio contents for assessment should follow the principles of best practice in qualitative research methodology. In particular attention should be paid to the concept of *trustworthiness*.

Effectiveness of portfolios

There are two BEME (best evidence medical and health professional education) reviews of the effectiveness of portfolios for learning and assessment. At the undergraduate level there is still limited evidence, but high-quality papers indicate that portfolios enhance student knowledge, self-awareness and engagement with reflection. However, portfolios are time intensive and students may only be motivated to complete them if they are assessed, and the quality of reflection is variable (Buckley *et al.*, 2009). Postgraduate portfolios appear to be practical and effective in enhancing personal responsibility for learning and for supporting professional development. Mentor feedback on content improves the efficacy, although many still remain sceptical particularly because of the time commitment. e-portfolios are more user friendly but there are concerns about the inter-rater reliability for summative assessments and it is recommended that other sources of data should also be used for summative judgments (Tochel *et al.*, 2009).

44 Setting pass marks

Practice points

- Standard setting uses a number of methods to set pass marks for written and practical skills assessments
- Most tests are criterion referenced, the score needed to pass the test is an absolute standard
- These are either test centred (focus is on judgement of the test content) or candidate centred (focus on judgements about individual learners)

Figure 44.1 Distribution of test marks amongst 250 candidates

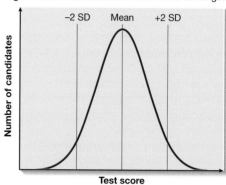

Table 44.1 Using Angoff's method for a 10-item test

Item	Judge 1	Judge 2	Judge 3	Judge 4	Judge 5	Judge 6	Judge 7	Judge 8	Min	Max	Range (highlight 20.4)	Judges mean
1	0.9	0.8	0.75	0.8	0.8	0.6	0.5	0.75	0.5	0.9	0.4	0.7
2	0.6	0.5	0.6	0.6	0.75	0.7	0.5	0.6	0.5	0.75	0.25	0.6
3	0.4	0.5	0.5	0.4	0.6	0.7	0.6	0.4	0.4	0.7	0.3	0.5
4	0.75	0.8	0.8	0.7	0.8	0.9	0.8	0.7	0.7	0.9	0.2	0.8
5	0.7	0.6	0.6	0.5	0.7	0.5	0.4	0.6	0.4	0.7	0.3	0.6
6	0.9	0.9	0.9	0.8	0.9	0.8	0.9	0.8	0.8	0.9	0.1	0.9
7	0.6	0.7	0.6	0.8	0.9	0.8	0.7	0.6	0.6	0.9	0.3	0.7
8	0.5	0.5	0.6	0.7	0.6	0.5	0.6	0.6	0.5	0.7	0.2	0.6
9	0.6	0.6	0.75	0.8	0.75	0.75	0.6	0.6	0.6	0.75	0.15	0.7
10	0.7	0.7	0.6	0.5	0.7	0.8	0.6	0.9	0.5	0.9	0.4	0.7
Overall means	0.7	0.7	0.7	0.7	0.8	0.7	0.6	0.7				0.7

Table 44.2 Using Ebel's method for a 60-item test

Category	Judge 1	Judge 2	Judge 3	Judge 4	Judge 5	Judge 6	Judge 7	Judge 8	Average proportion correct	No. questions	Expected score
EASY											
Must know	0.85	0.8	0.9	0.95	0.95	0.8	0.75	0.8	0.85	10	8.5
Good to know	0.7	0.7	0.75	0.75	0.6	0.65	0.65	0.65	0.68	10	6.8
Nice to know	0.6	0.6	0.65	0.6	0.65	0.6	0.6	0.55	0.61	10	6.1
HARD											
Must know	0.65	0.7	0.7	0.6	0.65	0.65	0.6	0.6	0.64	10	6.4
Good to know	0.55	0.55	0.6	0.55	0.6	0.5	0.5	0.55	0.55	10	5.5
Nice to know	0.4	0.45	0.4	0.4	0.4	0.45	0.4	0.4	0.41	10	4.1
STANDARD (cut score)											**37.4 out of 60**

Figure 44.2 Using the borderline regression method for an OSCE

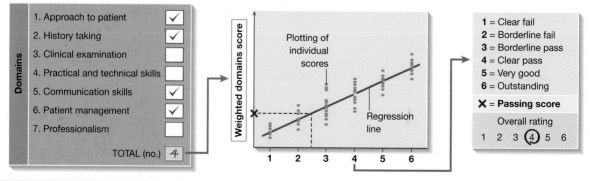

Medical Education at a Glance, First Edition. Edited by Judy McKimm, Kirsty Forrest and Jill Thistlethwaite © 2017 John Wiley & Sons, Ltd. Published 2017 by John Wiley & Sons, Ltd.

Whenever medical students or doctors in training take tests, some thought needs to be given to deciding what it takes to be 'good enough' to pass. Typically, candidates will achieve a range of scores, usually following a normal distribution, such as in Figure 44.1, with some doing very well, some very badly, and most in the middle. We need some idea of how to decide what an acceptable standard is: passing those who achieve it and failing those who do not.

In the 'old days', medical schools used to simply pass the top, for example, 90% of candidates in every test, or fail anyone more than two standard deviations below the mean. The performance of any one candidate was judged relative to the other candidates who took the same test, no matter what the overall level of the cohort was or the purpose of the test. This is called **norm referencing** and sets a relative standard. Whilst this is necessary in some cases, for example, for selection to limited places at medical school or into specialty training, there are obvious problems with this method when used to assess clinical competence. Capable candidates in a strong cohort might fail, even if they are clinically competent, and poor candidates might scrape through if the overall cohort is poor.

Clearly, patients and the public want to know that their doctor is competent and safe, and institutions want to pass everyone who meets this standard. In **criterion-referenced** assessment, the criteria for passing the test are decided in advance and the score that is needed to meet that standard is determined: an absolute standard. Everyone above that standard will pass. Most high-stakes medical assessments now use some form of criterion referencing, but there are a number of methods in use. Some of these are test centred and use judgements about the test content. Some are candidate centred and use judgements about individual candidates. All require some form of judgement.

Setting standards for written tests

There are a number of ways to set the pass mark for written tests. Two of the best known are the **Angoff** and **Ebel** methods, both of which are test centred and rely on human judges.

The Angoff method draws on a group of judges, usually five to ten, who work through all the items in the test and make a judgement about how hard they are for a hypothetical 'borderline' candidate. This is the candidate who is not clearly bad enough to fail, but also not clearly good enough to pass. They might be satisfactory in some areas, but poor in others. They might know the essential stuff fairly well, but not quite enough of other topics. Their knowledge is a bit patchy and their skills a bit 'hit and miss'. Conceptualising what this borderline candidate for this particular test looks like is a vital part of any Angoff group. Once this has been agreed, all judges look at all test items and estimate what proportion of a group of borderline candidates would get the item right. All scores are collected and the group discusses their judgements. Judges are able to change their estimates following the discussion. The estimates for each item are averaged to give the pass mark, as shown in Table 44.1. Sometimes, if the test has already been administered, judges can be shown the actual scores achieved for each question as a sort of reality check. The Angoff method is widely used around the world and there is good evidence for its reliability.

The Ebel method also begins with conceptualising the borderline candidate. Judges then classify the items in the test. For example, they might look at how easy or hard they are, or whether they represent core knowledge or more esoteric conditions. Once a classification table has been drawn up, all items are assigned a place in it. The judges then estimate the proportion of items in each group (e.g. core knowledge, medium difficulty) that the borderline candidate will get right. The allocations are discussed and judges can change their estimates. The pass mark is worked out from the average proportions and the number of items in each group, as shown in Table 44.2.

It is important that judges should be chosen who know the whole curriculum and what is expected of candidates. Both methods can be time consuming and logistically difficult to organise. All methods may be influenced by outliers: judges who hold extreme views ('hawks and doves'). Sometimes, decisions might have to be made by institutions about this, for example removing outlying judgements. Other statistical methods of quality assuring tests can look at reliability after the event and decisions may need to be taken about repeating, or adding to, standard setting judgements.

Setting standards for OSCEs

It is possible to use test-centred methods for OSCEs, but it is harder to estimate scores on OSCE stations, especially if domain-based marking is used (see Chapter 40). Candidate-centred methods use global judgements of candidate performance, collected by the examiners during the OSCE, to look at how the borderline group of candidates did. In the borderline regression method, individual station scores are plotted out and statistically regressed against the global scores, using a computer programme, and the **cut-off score** is read off to give the pass mark for the station (Figure 44.2).

The number of points on the global rating and what they mean will be determined in advance when stations are written, along with where to read off the cut score. Other measures may also be used to determine whether candidates pass the overall OSCE, such as passing a certain percentage of stations overall or passing a number of 'essential' stations.

Every method of setting a pass mark is a judgement and no method is perfect. However, they all aim to adequately give a boundary between candidates who achieve the predetermined standard and those who do not.

45 Developing yourself as a medical educator

Figure 45.1 The teacher–researcher continuum

A number of writers have described the roles of the medical educator as lying on a continuum from teaching to research (e.g. Fincher and Work, 2006); others include management and/or leadership (e.g. Bligh and Brice, 2009). The figure below summarises the continuum.

Excellent teaching	Scholarly teaching	Scholarly teaching	Scholarship of teaching	Research	Professional activities
Designs and implements activities to improve learning	Utilises knowledge and theory to enhance practice	Uses literature and tools to evaluate teaching with peer-review	Peer-reviewed and publicly disseminated product that others can use	Carries out original research that increases or expands knowledge	e.g. management, leadership, citizenship. Scholarly, evidence based approach to improving services, organisations and systems

Figure 45.2 Developing your educator practice

In this figure, we have adapted the model in Figure 45.1 in terms of how educators might engage with different activities along the continuum. It summarises some of the knowledge, skills and activities individuals might need to acquire and engage in as they develop their educational practice.

Excellent teaching	Scholarly teaching	Scholarly teaching	Scholarship of teaching	Research	Professional activities
Teaching and facilitation skills, assessor skills. Understanding of context, curriculum etc	Knowledge acquisition, applies theory to practice	Evaluation skills, subjects self to peer review	Develops educational products, disseminates via e.g. conference presentations, journal articles, books	Research skills, masters/PhD programme. Collaboration	Engagement in socially accountable management and leadership activities of initiatives, projects, curricula, departments, organisations, services

Figure 45.3 Academy of Medical Educators' Professional Standards Framework. Source: Reproduced with permission from AoME.

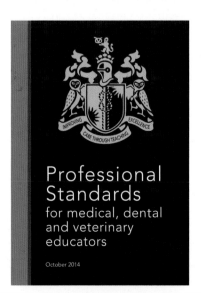

Medical Education at a Glance, First Edition. Edited by Judy McKimm, Kirsty Forrest and Jill Thistlethwaite © 2017 John Wiley & Sons, Ltd. Published 2017 by John Wiley & Sons, Ltd.

Medical education is becoming increasingly *professionalised* with education organisations being required to deliver, the body of knowledge and the opportunities for engagement, development and advancement. Medical education is, however, a very broad discipline and, given the wide range of people involved, professional development opportunities and activities are extensive and can be tailored to stage of learning or career. When planning development activities, it is helpful to consider where you (and your interests) lie on the *teaching–research continuum* (Fincher and Work, 2006) (Figure 45.1). Figure 45.2 illustrates some of the activities, skills and knowledge that might help develop your educational practice. We expand these ideas in the rest of the chapter.

Of course, all professionals need to keep up to date with and extend their understanding of their subject through reading books and journals, but the focus of this chapter is on other ways of developing as an educator. The main purpose of educational development is to provide the best medical education we can, within the context in which we work and so most people will dip in and out of formal professional development activities throughout their lives, depending on their needs.

Development activities

Short courses and workshops

An obvious starting point for developing your educator practice is to attend workshops, take courses or undertake a degree programme in general, medical or health professions' education. These might be offered by universities, postgraduate centres or organisations, professional bodies (e.g. Medical Royal Colleges or Medical Councils), health providers or private providers. Depending on your stage of training or career or your educational role, some educational courses may be mandatory. For example in the UK, if you are a university lecturer or educational supervisor, you are required to undertake certain approved courses, some of which are externally accredited. These are primarily geared towards improving practical teaching or assessment skills. However, for those more involved in education, developing scholarly teaching (i.e. practice grounded in theory (Bligh and Brice, 2009) might be required (Figure 45.1).

Depending on your role and interest, a wide range of other courses (online as well as face to face) are available, which cover many of the topics in this book. Having a knowledge base and understanding of educational principles and terminology not only gives you more confidence and credibility in educational settings but also should equip you to deliver higher-quality education.

Degree programmes

Many medical schools now include education as part of the core curriculum and some provide opportunities for students to intercalate a medical education degree. Increasingly, doctors in training are able to apply for educational-oriented programmes, some with time out for a specific role (e.g. teaching fellow) or to study for a postgraduate award. A large number of masters' programmes are available around the world in both face-to-face or distance learning modalities. Typical core content areas that masters' and other courses cover in the early stages include: curriculum design; learning theories; teaching methods; assessment methods and evaluation (or quality assurance). Some programmes also include peer-observed and/or assessed teaching practice. For those progressing to masters' dissertation, you will also learn about research methods and design a research study. This starts to move you along the teaching–research continuum, and you might go further by

undertaking a PhD or other doctoral programme which allows you to research in depth about a topic.

Experience and practice

Another way of developing your practice is to gain experience in education through offering to work on projects or initiatives, these might be internal or external to your organisation. Working with experienced colleagues is an excellent way to learn about the realities of medical education and apply some of the theory to actual practice. For those interested in educational management or leadership, this is essential and this is where a mentor or coach might be helpful (see Chapters 33 and 34). Engagement in professional activities such as these, which may be at all levels (see Figure 45.2) may well require further development in management, leadership or entrepreneurship, which again can be done through a number of different ways.

Associations

A number of associations dedicated to medical or health professions' education exist around the world which are an invaluable resource for your development. Many provide opportunities for participation in face-to-face or online activities (such as webinars) and most welcome members from various countries, contexts or professions. Local or national organisations may have regular meetings or groups on specific topics (e.g. simulation, assessment, selection) whereas larger regional organisations usually have an annual conference or meeting. These are excellent venues for networking, meeting like-minded colleagues, hearing from experts in their field and presenting your work. Conferences usually have pre- and intraconference workshops on various topics, both on general education and specific topics. Some associations also provide free or reduced rate access to educational resources, such as journals, educational guides and online courses or webinars.

Research and publication

Whilst many educators will focus primarily on their teaching practice or educational management or leadership, others will be more interested in actively engaging in research to improve educational practice. Whether you are involved in evaluation–type activities or a large research project, identifying how and where you might disseminate your work is important. Most educators start off presenting locally, then moving to larger national or regional conferences prior to writing for publication, but this largely depends on your research and who you are working with. Learning to write or present well is often a process of trial and error, it takes practice and you need constructive feedback. Experienced colleagues and mentors can again be invaluable in providing guidance, advice and support.

Professional recognition

Whilst medical education associations have long welcomed members on a subscription basis, a relatively recent development in university and professional education is the establishment of professional standards for both individual educators and for programmes (for example Figure 45.3). This development provides opportunities for educators to obtain formal professional recognition of their achievements in education. Recognition typically involves either successful completion of an accredited programme or an individual application summarising achievements and impact in various educational domains, reflection (demonstrating values), evidence and referee support. Recognition is usually awarded at various levels, reflecting the experience, activities and impact of the educator.

Further reading

Part 1 Overview and broad concepts

Chapters 1 and 2 About medical education

Bleakley A, Bligh J, Browne J (2011) *Medical Education for the Future: Identity, Power and Location.* Springer, London.

Calman KC (2007) *Medical Education: Past, Present and Future.* Churchill Livingstone/Elsevier, Philadelphia.

Cavenagh P, Leinster SJ, Miles S (2011) (eds) *The Changing Face of Medical Education.* Radcliffe Publishing, Abingdon.

Dent J, Harden RM (eds) (2017) *A Practical Guide for Medical Teachers.* 5th edition, Elsevier Health Sciences.

Swanwick T (ed) (2014) *Understanding Medical Education: Evidence, theory and practice,* 2nd edn. Wiley and the Association of Medical Education, Chichester.

Walsh K (ed) (2013) *Oxford Textbook of Medical Education.* Oxford University Press, Oxford.

Wijnen-Meijer M, Burdick W, Alofs L, *et al.* (2013) Stages and transitions in medical education around the world: clarifying structures and terminology. *Medical Teacher,* 35, 301–307.

Chapter 3 Evidence-guided education

Cleland J, Durning SJ (eds) (2015) *Researching Medical Education.* Wiley-Blackwell, Chichester.

Grant MJ, Booth A (2009) A typology of reviews: an analysis of 14 review types and associated methodologies. *Health Information and Libraries Journal,* 26, 91–108.

Hope D, Dewar A (2015) Conducting quantitative educational research: a short guide for clinical teachers. *The Clinical Teacher,* 12, 299–304.

Somekh B, Lewin C (eds) (2005) *Research Methods in the Social Sciences.* Sage, London.

Tai J, Ajjawi R (2016) Undertaking and reporting qualitative research. *The Clinical Teacher,* 13, 175–182.

Chapters 4 and 5 Learning theories

Bleakley A (2013) Working in "teams" in an era of "liquid" healthcare: What is the use of theory? *Journal of Interprofessional Care,* 27, 18–26.

Bleakley A, Bligh J, Browne J (2011) *Medical Education for the Future: Identity, Power and Location.* Springer, Dordrecht.

Chen HC, Cate O, O'Sullivan P, *et al.* (2016) Students' goal orientations, perceptions of early clinical experiences and learning outcomes. *Medical Education,* 50, 203–213.

Cook V, Daly C, Newman M (eds) (2012) *Work-Based Learning in Clinical Settings – Insights from Socio-Cultural Perspectives.* Radcliffe, Oxford.

Kaufman DM (2010) Applying educational theory in practice. In: Cantillon P, Wood D (eds) *ABC of Learning and Teaching in Medicine,* 2nd edn. Blackwell Publishing Ltd, pp. 1–5.

Knowles M, Holton E, Swanson R (2005) *The Adult Learner.* Elsevier, Burlington, MA.

Lee A, Dunston R (2011) Practice, learning and change: Towards a retheorisation of professional education. *Teaching in Higher Education,* 16, 483–494.

Malloch M, Cairns L, Evans K, O'Connor B (2011) *The Sage Handbook of Workplace Learning.* Sage, London.

Orsini C, Binnie VI, Wilson SL (2016) Determinants and outcomes of motivation in health professions' education: a systematic review based on self-determination theory. *Journal of Educational Evaluation for Health Professions,* 13, 19.

Smith MK (1999) *Learning Theory. The Encyclopedia of Informal Education.* Available at: www.infed.org/biblio/b-learn.htm (accessed August 2016).

Torre DM, Daley BJ, Sebastian JL, Elnicki DM (2006) Overview of current learning theories for medical educators. *American Journal of Medicine,* 119, 903–907.

Wearn A, O'Callaghan A, Barrow M (2016) Becoming a different doctor. In: Land R, Meyer JHF, Flanagan MT (eds) *Threshold Concepts in Practice.* Sense Publishers, pp. 223–238.

Chapters 6 and 7 Curriculum, planning and design

Barrott J, Sunderland AB, Micklin JP, McKenzie Smith M (2013) Designing effective simulation activities. In: Forrest K, McKimm J, Edgar S (eds). *Essential Simulation in Clinical Education.* Wiley Blackwell, Chichester, pp. 168–195.

Burgess AW, McGregor DM, Mellis CM (2014) Applying established guidelines to team-based learning programs in medical schools: a systematic review. *Academic Medicine,* 89, 678–688.

Cooke M, Irby DM, Sullivan W, Ludmerer KM (2006) American medical education 100 years after the Flexner report. *New England Journal of Medicine,* 355, 1339–1344.

Frank JR, Danoff D (2007) The CanMEDS initiative: implementing an outcomes-based framework of physician competencies. *Medical Teacher,* 29, 642–647.

Harden RM (1999) AMEE Guide No. 14: Outcome-based education: Parts 1–5. *Medical Teacher,* 21, 1–6.

Jones R, Higgs R, de Angelis C, Prideaux D (2001) Changing face of medical curricula. *Lancet,* 357(9257), 699–703.

Lake FR, Ryan G. (2004) Teaching on the run tip 3: planning a teaching episode. *Medical Journal of Australia,* 180, 643–644.

Prideaux D (2007) Curriculum development in medical education: from acronyms to dynamism. *Teaching and Teacher Education,* 23, 294–302.

Learning Theories. Available at: www.learning-theories.com [A website all about learning theories explains more about the underpinnings of curriculum design and philosophy.]

INFED. Available at: www.infed.org (accessed Oct. 2016). [INFED is another useful general site that covers many aspects of education, learning and community.]

Chapter 8 Equality, diversity and inclusivity

Equality and Diversity UK (2011) *Embedding Equality and Diversity into Every Day Practice: Post-16 Education Toolkit.* Available at: www.equalityanddiversity.co.uk/samples/sample-embedding-equality-and-diversity-into-everyday-practice.pdf (accessed 16 May 2016).

McKimm J, Da Silva AS, Edwards S, *et al.* (2015) Women and leadership in medicine and medical education: international perspectives. In: *Gender, Careers and Inequalities in Medicine and Medical Education: International Perspectives.* Emerald Group Publishing Limited, pp. 69–98.

Chapter 9 Principles of selection

Patterson F, Knight A, Dowell J, *et al.* (2016) How effective are selection methods in medical education? A systematic review. *Medical Education*, 50, 36–60.

Powis D (2015) Selecting medical students: An unresolved challenge. *Medical Teacher*, 37, 252–260.

Sladek RM, Bond MJ, Frost LK, Prior KN (2016) Predicting success in medical school: a longitudinal study of common Australian student selection tools. *BMC Medical Education*, 16, 1.

White J, Brownell K, Lemay JF, Lockyer JM (2012) "What Do They Want Me To Say?" The hidden curriculum at work in the medical school selection process: a qualitative study. *BMC Medical Education*, 12, 1.

Chapter 10 Evaluation

King JA, Stevahn L (2013) *Interactive evaluation practice. Mastering the interpersonal dynamics of program evaluation.* Sage, Los Angeles

Chapter 11 Educational leadership

Eagly AH, Heilman ME (2016) Gender and leadership: Introduction to the special issue. *Leadership Quarterly*, 3, 349–353.

Earis J, Garner J, Haddock D, Jha V (2016) Medical students learn about leadership from the army. *Medical Education*, 50, 568–569.

Gorsky D, MacLeod A (2016) Shifting norms and expectations for medical school leaders: a textual analysis of career advertisements 2000–2004 cf. 2010–2014. *Journal of Higher Education Policy and Management*, 38, 5–18.

Lumb A, Murdoch-Eaton D (2014) Electives in undergraduate medical education: AMEE Guide No. 88. *Medical Teacher*, 36, 557–572.

McKimm J, Cotton P, Garden A, Needham G (2013) Educational leadership. In: Walsh K (ed) *Oxford Textbook of Medical Education.* Oxford University Press, Oxford, pp. 722–736.

McKimm J, Lieff SJ (2013) Medical education leadership. In: Dent J, Harden RM (eds) *A Practical Guide for Medical Teachers.* Elsevier Health Sciences, pp. 343–352.

McKimm J, Swanwick T (2014) Educational leadership. In: Swanwick T (ed) *Understanding Medical Education: Evidence, Theory and Practice,* 2nd edn. ASME/Wiley Blackwell, Chichester, pp. 473–492.

Shapiro JP, Stefkovich JA (2016) *Ethical leadership and decision making in education: Applying theoretical perspectives to complex dilemmas.* Routledge, London.

Souba WW (2016) Resilience-back to the future. *JAMA Surgery,* 151, 896–897.

Storey J (ed) (2016) *Leadership in Organizations: Current Issues and Key Trends.* Routledge, London.

Chapter 12 International perspectives

Al-Eraky MM, Donkers J, Wajid G, van Merrienboer JJG (2014) A Delphi study of medical professionalism in Arabian countries: the Four-Gates model. *Medical Teacher*, 36, S8–S16.

Ho MJ, Shaw K, Liu TH, *et al.* (2015) Equal, global, local: discourses in Taiwan's international medical graduate debate. *Medical education*, 49, 48–59.

Roland M, Rao SR, Sibbald B, *et al.* (2011) Professional values and reported behaviours of doctors in the USA and UK: quantitative survey. *BMJ Quality and Safety,* 20, 515–521.

Part 2 Medical education in practice

Chapters 13 and 14 Large group teaching

Bligh DA (2000) *What's the Use of Lectures?* Jossey-Bass, San Francisco, CA.

Brown G, Manogue M (2001) AMEE Medical Education Guide No 22: refreshing lecturing: a guide for lecturers. *Medical Teacher,* 23, 231–244.

Dornan T, Ellaway RH (2011) Teaching and learning in large groups: lecturing in the twenty-first century. In: Dornan T, Mann KV, Scherpbier AJ, Spencer J (eds) *Medical Education Theory and Practice.* Churchill Livingstone/Elsevier, Edinburgh, pp. 157–170.

Long A, Lock B (2014) Lectures and large groups. In: Swanwick T (ed) *Understanding Medical Education: Evidence, Theory and Practice,* 2nd edn. ASME/Wiley Blackwell, Chichester, pp. 137–148.

McKimm J (2014) *Improve your Lecturing.* NHS Health Education Central, East, North West and South London. Available at: www.faculty.londondeanery.ac.uk/e-learning/improve-your-lecturing-1 (accessed August 2016).

Chapters 15 and 16 Small group teaching

Dennick R, Spencer J (2011) Teaching and learning in small groups. In: Dornan T, Mann KV, Scherpbier AJ, Spencer J (eds), *Medical Education Theory and Practice.* Churchill Livingstone/Elsevier, Edinburgh, pp. 131–156.

McCrorie P (2014) Teaching and leading small groups. In: Swanwick T (ed) *Understanding Medical Education: Evidence, theory and practice,* 2nd edn. Wiley and the Association of Medical Education, Chichester, pp. 123–136.

Chapters 17 and 18 Clinical teaching

Billet S (2004) Workplace participatory practices: conceptualising workplaces as learning environments. *Journal of Workplace Learning,* 16, 312–324.

Health Talk. Available at: www.healthtalkonline.org (accessed August 2016). [Based on qualitative research into patient experiences, led by Oxford University researchers. Includes personal stories about health and illness from a wide range of service users.]

Irby D, Wilkerson L (2008) Teaching when time is limited. *British Medical Journal*, 336, 384–387.

Lake F, Hamdorf J (2004) Teaching on the run tip no. 5: teaching a skill. *Medical Journal of Australia,* 181: 327–328.

Lake F, Ryan G (2004) Teaching on the run tip no 4: teaching with patients. *Medical Journal of Australia,* 181, 158–159.

Lake F, Vickery A (2006) Teaching on the run tip no 14: teaching in ambulatory care. *Medical Journal of Australia,* 185, 166–167.

McKimm J (2014) *Involving Patients in Health Professions' Education.* Available at: www.faculty.londondeanery.ac.uk/e-learning/involving-patients-in-health-professions-education (accessed August 2016).

Morris C, McKimm J (2014) *Facilitating Learning in the Workplace.* Available at: www.faculty.londondeanery.ac.uk/e-learning/facilitating-learning-in-the-workplace-1 (accessed August 2016).

Patient Voices. Available at: www.patientvoices.org.uk (accessed August 2016). [Provides over 100 digital stories from patients, carers and health workers on a range of topics.]

Spencer JA, Godolphin W, Karpenko N, Towle A (2011) *Can Patients be Teachers? Involving Patients and Service Users in Health Professions' Education.* Report to The Health Foundation, October 2011.

Swanwick T (2005) Informal learning in postgraduate medical education: from cognitivism to 'culturism'. *Medical Education,* 39, 859–865.

Chapters 19 and 20 Simulation

Bligh D, Bleakley, A (2006) Distributing menus to hungry learners: can learning by simulation become simulation of learning? *Medical Teacher,* 28, 606–613.

Cleland JA, Abe K, Rethans J (2009) The use of simulated patients in medical education: AMEE Guide No 42. *Medical Teacher,* 31, 477–486.

Cumin D, Merry AF, Weller JM (2008) Standards for simulation. *Anaesthesia,* 63, 1281–1287.

Forrest K, McKimm J (2014) *Simulation in Health Professions' Education.* Available at: www.faculty.londondeanery.ac.uk/e-learning/simulation-in-health-professions-education (accessed August 2016).

Forrest K, McKimm J, Edgar S (eds) (2013) *Essential Simulation in Clinical Education.* Wiley Blackwell, Chichester.

Khan K, Pattison T, Sherwood M (2011) Simulation in medical education. *Medical Teacher,* 33, 1–3.

Motola I, Devine LA, Chung HS, *et al.* (2013) Simulation in healthcare education: a best evidence practical guide. AMEE Guide No. 82. *Medical Teacher,* 35, e1511–e1530.

Nestel D, Groom J, Eikeland-Husebo S, *et al.* (2011) Does simulation-based medical education with deliberate practice yield better results than traditional clinical education? A meta-analytic comparative review of the evidence. *Academic Medicine,* 86, 706–711.

Chapter 21 Patient involvement

Towle A, Farrell C, Gaines M *et al.* (2016) The patient's voice in health and social care professional education. The Vancouver Statement. *International Journal of Health Governance,* 2, 1–6.

Chapter 22 Ward-based and bedside teaching

Ker J (2008) Teaching on a ward round. *BMJ,* 337, a1930.

Monrouxe L, Rees CE, Bradley P (2009) The construction of patients' involvement in hospital bedside encounters. *Qualitative Health Research,* 19, 918–930.

Peters M, ten Cate O (2014) Bedside teaching in medical education: a literature review. *Perspectives in Medical Education,* 3, 76–88.

Williams K, Ramani S, Fraser B, Orlander J (2008) Improving bedside teaching: Findings from a focus group study of learners. *Academic Medicine,* 83, 257–264.

Woodley N, McKelvie K, Kellett C (2016) Bedside teaching: specialists versus non-specialists. *The Clinical Teacher,* 13, 138–141.

Chapter 23 Learning and teaching in ambulatory settings

Christensen S, Thistlethwaite JE (2009) Medical students in primary care: helping teachers enhance their teaching. *Clinical Teacher,* 6, 225–228.

Mehay R (2012) *The Essential Handbook for GP Training and Education.* Radcliffe Publishing, London.

Sprake C, Cantillon P, Metcalf J, Spencer J (2008) Teaching in ambulatory care. *BMJ,* 337, 690–692.

Thistlethwaite JE, Bartle E, Chong AL, *et al.* (2013) A review of longitudinal community and hospital placements in medical education: BEME Guide No. 26. *Medical Teacher,* 35, e1340–e1364.

Thistlethwaite JE, Hudson J, Kidd M (2007) Moving more of the medical curriculum into the community. *The Clinical Teacher,* 4, 232–237.

Chapter 24 Teaching in the operating theatre

Carley S, Morris H, Kilroy D (2007) Clinical teaching in emergency medicine: the board round at Hope Hospital emergency department. *Emergency Medicine Journal,* 24, 659–661.

Murji A, Luketic L, Sobel ML, *et al.* (2016) Evaluating the effect of distractions in the operating room on clinical decision-making and patient safety. *Surgical Endoscopy,* 30, 4499–4504.

Vinden C, Malthaner R, McGee R, *et al.* (2016) Teaching surgery takes time: the impact of surgical education on time in the operating room. *Canadian Journal of Surgery,* 59, 87.

Chapter 25 Interprofessional education

Forman D, Jones M, Thistlethwaite JE (eds) (2014) *Leadership Development for Interprofessional Education and Practice.* Palgrave, Basingstoke.

Stone J (2010) Moving interprofessional learning forward through formal assessment. *Medical Education,* 44, 396–403.

Thistlethwaite JE (2012) Interprofessional education: a review of context, learning and the research agenda. *Medical Education,* 46, 58–70.

Examples of IPE competency frameworks:

Canadian Interprofessional Health Collaborative (2010) CIHC. Available at: www.cihc.ca/files/CIHC_IPCompetencies_Feb1210.pdf (accessed August 2016).

Interprofessional Education Collaborative Expert Panel (IPEC) (2011) Available at: www.aacn.nche.edu/education-resources/ipecreport.pdf (accessed August 2016).

Thistlethwaite JE, Forman D, Rogers G, *et al.* (2014). Interprofessional education competencies and frameworks in health: A comparative analysis. *Academic Medicine,* 89, 869–874.

Chapter 26 Reflective practice

Grant A, McKimm J, Murphy F. *Developing Reflective Practice: A Guide for Medical Students, Doctors and Teachers.* Wiley, Chichester (in press).

Kember D (2001) *Reflective Teaching and Learning in the Health Professions.* Blackwell Science, Oxford.

Nguyen QD, Fernandez N, Karsenti T, Charlin B (2014) What is reflection? A conceptual analysis of major definitions and a proposal of a five-component model. *Medical Education,* 12, 1176–1189.

Sandars J (2009) The use of reflection in medical education. AMEE guide No.44. *Medical Teacher,* 8, 685–695.

Chapter 27 Teaching clinical reasoning

Clinical Reasoning. Available at: www.clinical-reasoning.org (accessed Oct. 2016).

Cooper N, Frain J (eds) (2016) *ABC of Clinical Reasoning.* Wiley Blackwell, Chichester.

Croskerry P (2014) Bias: a normal operating characteristic of the diagnosing brain. *Diagnosis,* 1, 23–27.

Croskerry P, Nimmo GR (2011) Better clinical decision making and reducing diagnostic error. *Journal of the Royal Collage of Physicians Edinburgh,* 41, 155–162.

JAMA Rational Clinical Examination Series. Available at: http://jama.jamanetwork.com/collection.aspx?categoryid=6257 (accessed August 2016).

McGee SR (2007) *Evidence Based Physical Diagnosis,* 3rd edn. Elsevier Saunders, Philadelphia.

Trowbridge RL, Rencic JJ, Durning SJ (eds) (2015) *Teaching Clinical Reasoning.* American College of Physicians, Philadelphia.

Chapter 28 Professionalism

Cruess RL, Cruess SR, Steinert Y (eds) (2016) *Teaching Medical Professionalism. Supporting the Development of a Professional Identity.* Cambridge Medicine, Cambridge.

Thistlethwaite JE, McKimm J (2015) *Professionalism at a Glance.* Wiley-Backwell, Chichester.

Chapter 29 Peer teaching

Iwata K, Furmedge DS (2016) Are all peer tutors and their tutoring really effective? Considering quality assurance. *Medical Education,* 50, 395–397.

Chapter 30 Communication

Iedema R, Piper D, Manidis M (2015) *Communicating Quality and Safety in Health Care.* Cambridge University Press, Cambridge. [Text primarily for learners but well referenced and has many practical examples for facilitators.]

Chapter 31 Problem-based and case-based learning

Albanese M, Dast LA (2013) Problem-based learning. In: Walsh K (ed) *The Oxford Textbook of Medical Education.* Oxford University Press, Oxford, pp. 25–37.

Albanese M, Dast LA (2014) Problems-based learning. In: Swanwick T (ed) *Understanding Medical Education: Evidence, Theory and Practice,* 2nd edn. Wiley and the Association of Medical Education, Chichester, pp. 63–80.

Sefton AE, Frommer M (2013) Problem-based learning. In: Dent J, Harden R (eds) *A Practical Guide for Medical Teachers,* 4th edn. Churchill Livingstone/Elsevier Ltd, London, pp. 166–172.

Chapter 32 Learner support

Duvivier RJ, Dent J (2013) Student support. In: Dent J, Harden R (eds) *A Practical Guide for Medical Teachers,* 4th edn. Churchill Livingstone/Elsevier Ltd, London, pp. 362–368.

Chapter 33 Professional development and performance management

General Medical Council (2012) *Continuing Professional Development: Guidance for All Doctors.* Available at: www.gmc-uk.org/Continuing_professional_development_guidance_for_all_doctors_0316.pdf_56438625.pdf (accessed August 2016).

General Medical Council (2010) *The Effectiveness of Continuing Professional Development.* Available at: www.gmc-uk.org/Effectiveness_of_CPD_Final_Report.pdf_34306281.pdf (accessed August 2016).

Academy of Medical Educators (2014) *Professional Standards for Medical, Dental and Veterinary Educators.* Available at: www.medicaleducators.org/write/MediaManager/AOME_Professional_Standards_2014.pdf (accessed August 2016).

Van Dooren W, Bouckaert G, Halligan J (2015) *Performance Management in the Public Sector.* Routledge, London.

Chapter 34 Mentoring and supervision

Chartered Institute of Personnel and Development. Available at: www.cipd.co.uk/hr-resources/factsheets/coaching-mentoring.aspx (accessed Oct. 2016). [More on the difference between coaching and mentoring.]

Cooper N, Forrest K (2009) *Essential Guide to Educational Supervision in Postgraduate Medical Education.* Wiley Blackwell/BMJ books, Chichester.

Sambunjak D, Straus SE, Marušić A (2006) Mentoring in academic medicine: a systematic review. *JAMA,* 296, 1103–1115.

Viney R, McKimm J (2010) Mentoring. *British Journal of Hospital Medicine,* 71, 106–109.

Chapters 35 and 36 Social media

Benfield G, De Laat M (2010) Collaborative knowledge building. In: Sharpe R, Beetham H, de Freitas S (eds) *Rethinking Learning for a Digital Age: How Learners Are Shaping Their Own Experiences.* Routledge, New York, pp. 184–198.

Facer K, Selwyn N (2010) *Social Networking: Key Messages From the Research.* In: Sharpe R, Beetham H, de Freitas S (eds) *Rethinking Learning for a Digital Age: How Learners Are Shaping Their Own Experiences.* Routledge, New York, pp. 31–42.

Henderson M (2015) *Using social media: assumptions, challenges and risks.* In: Henderson MJ, Romeo G (eds) *Teaching and Digital Technologies: Big Issues and Critical Questions.* Cambridge University Press, Cambridge, Port Melbourne, Vic, pp. 115–126.

JISC. Available at: https://www.jisc.ac.uk/guides (accessed Oct. 2016). [A series of guides are available from JISC on various topics related to social media including selecting technologies and safeguarding learners online.]

Part 3 Assessment and feedback

Chapter 37 Feedback

Boud D, Molloy E (eds) (2013) *Feedback in Higher Education: Understanding it and Doing it Well.* Routledge, Abingdon.

McKimm J (2016) *Effective Feedback.* Health Education North Central and East, South and North West London Faculty Development module. Available at: www.faculty.londondeanery.ac.uk/e-learning/effective-feedback (accessed August 2016).

Race P (2016) *Using Feedback to Help Students Learn.* Higher Education Academy, York. Available at: http://wap.rdg.ac.uk/web/FILES/EngageinFeedback/Race_using_feedback_to_help_students_learn.pdf (accessed August 2016).

Chapter 38 Principles of assessment

Norman, G (2014) When I say…reliability. *Medical Education,* 48, 946–947.

Chapter 39 Written assessment

Campbell DE (2011) How to write good multiple-choice questions. *Journal of Paediatrics and Child Health*, 47, 322–325.

Case SM, Swanson DB (2002) *Item Writing Manual,* 3rd edn. NBME, Philadelphia. Available at: www.nbme.org/publications/item-writing-manual-download.html (accessed August 2016).

Haladyna TM, Rodriguez MC (2013) *Developing and Validating Test Items.* Routledge, London.

Schuwirth LWT, van der Vleuten CPM (2004) Different written assessment methods: what can be said about their strengths and weaknesses? *Medical Education*, 38, 974–979.

Chapter 40 Clinical skills assessment

Harden RM (2016) Revisiting 'assessment of clinical competence using an objective structured clinical examination (OSCE). *Medical Education*, 50, 376–379.

Harden RM, Lilley P. Patricio M (2015) *The Definitive Guide to the OSCE: The Objective Structured Clinical Examination as a Performance Assessment.* Elsevier, Edinburgh.

Hodges BD, Lingard L (eds) (2012) *The Question of Competence: Reconsidering Medical Education in the Twenty-first Century.* Cornell University Press, USA.

Chapter 41 Work-based assessment

Govaerts M. ven der Vleuten CPM (2013) Validity in work-based assessment: expanding our horizons. *Medical Education*, 47, 1164–1174.

Chapter 42 Assessing professionalism

Cruess RL, Cruess SR, Steinert Y (2016) Amending Miller's pyramid to include professional identity formation. *Academic Medicine*, 91, 180–185.

Guraya SY, Guraya SS, Mahabbat NA, *et al.* (2016) The desired concept maps and goal setting for assessing professionalism in medicine. *Journal of Clinical and Diagnostic Research,* 10, JE01–JE05.

Hughes LJ, Mitchell M, Johnston AN (2016) 'Failure to fail' in nursing–A catch phrase or a real issue? A systematic integrative literature review. *Nurse Education in Practice*, 20, 54–63.

Lynch DC, Surdyk PM, Eiser AR (2004) Assessing professionalism: a review of the literature. *Medical Teacher*, 26, 366–373.

McConnell MM, Harms S, Saperson K (2016) Meaningful feedback in medical education: challenging the "failure to fail" using narrative methodology. *Academic Psychiatry*, 40, 377–379.

Nixon LJ, Gladding SP, Duffy BL (2016) Describing failure in a clinical clerkship: implications for identification, assessment and remediation for struggling learners. *Journal of General Internal Medicine*, 31, 1172–1179.

Parker M (2006) Assessing professionalism: theory and practice. *Medical Teacher*, 28, 399–403.

Stern DT (2006) *Measuring Medical Professionalism.* Oxford University Press.

Wilkinson TJ, Wade WB, Knock LD (2009) A blueprint to assess professionalism: results of a systematic review. *Academic Medicine*, 84, 551–558.

Chapter 43 Portfolios

Davis M, McKimm J, Forrest K (2013) Portfolios. In: *How to Assess Doctors and Health Professionals.* Wiley Blackwell/BMJ Books, Chichester, pp. 68–80.

Chapter 44 Setting pass marks

De Champlain AF (2014) Standard setting methods in medical education. In: Swanwick T (ed) *Understanding Medical Education: Evidence, Theory and Practice*, ASME/ Wiley Blackwell, Chichester, pp. 305–316.

McKinley DW, Norcini J (2013) Setting standards. In: Walsh K (ed) *Oxford Textbook of Medical Education.* Oxford University Press, Oxford, pp. 421–431.

Norcini J, McKinley DW (2013) Standard setting. In Dent J, Harden R, Hodges B (eds) *A Practical Guide for Medical Teachers.* Churchill Livingstone, London, pp. 292–306.

Chapter 45 Developing yourself as a medical educator

Bertram A, Yeh HC, Bass EB, *et al.* (2015) How we developed the GIM clinician–educator mentoring and scholarship program to assist faculty with promotion and scholarly work. *Medical Teacher*, 37, 131–135.

Schwartz A, Young R, Hicks PJ, (2016) Medical education practice-based research networks: Facilitating collaborative research. *Medical Teacher*, 38, 64–74.

Simpson D, Sullivan, GM (2015) Knowledge translation for education journals in the digital age. *Journal of Graduate Medical Education*, 7, 315–317.

Steinert Y (ed) (2014) *Faculty Development in the Health Professions.* Springer Netherlands.

Swanwick T, McKimm J (2010) Professional development of medical educators. *British Journal of Hospital Medicine,* 71, 164–168.

Many medical education journals are available, which include:

Academic Medicine. This is the journal of the Association of American Medical Colleges. Available at: http://journals.lww.com/academicmedicine/pages/default.aspx (accessed August 2016).

Medical Education. This and *The Clinical Teacher* are the journals of ASME (Association for the Study of Medical Education). Available at: http://onlinelibrary.wiley.com/journal/10.1111/(ISSN) 1365-2923 and http://onlinelibrary.wiley.com/journal/10.1111/(ISSN)1743-498X (accessed August 2016).

Medical Teacher. This is the journal of AMEE, the Association for Medical Education in Europe. Available at: www.medicalteacher.org (accessed August 2016).

Many other associations have their own journals, as do some medical colleges and universities.

References

Academy of Medical Educators (2014) *Professional Standards for Medical, Dental and Veterinary Educators.* Available at: www.medicaleducators.org (accessed August 2016).

Amin Z (2012) Purposeful assessment. *Medical Education,* 46, 4–7.

Australian Medical Council (2012) Available at: www.amc.org.au/files/d0ffcecda9608cf49c66c93a79a4ad549638bea0_original.pdf (accessed Oct. 2016).

Banchi H, Bell R (2008) The many levels of inquiry-based learning. *Science and Children,* 46, 26–29.

Bandura A (1977) *Social Learning Theory.* Prentice-Hall, Oxford, England.

Barr H, Freeth D, Hammick M, *et al.* (2000) *Evaluations for Interprofessional Education. A United Kingdom Review for Health and Social Care.* CAIPE/BERA, London.

Barr H, Hammick M, Koppel I, Reeves S (1999) Evaluating interprofessional education: Two systematic reviews for health and social care. *British Educational Research Journal,* 25, 533–543.

Barr H, Koppel I, Reeves S, *et al.* (2005) *Effective Interprofessional Education. Argument, Assumption and Evidence.* Blackwell Publishing, Oxford.

Barrow M, McKimm J, Gasquoine S, Rowe D. (2015) Collaborating in healthcare delivery: exploring conceptual differences at the "bedside". *Journal of Interprofessional Care,* 29, 119–124.

Barrows H, Tamblyn R (1980) *Problem-based Learning: An Approach to Medical Education.* Springer, New York.

Becher T, Trowler PR (2001) *Academic Tribes and Territories.* Society for Research in Higher Education, Buckingham.

Biggs J (1999) *Teaching for Quality Learning at University.* SRHE and Open University Press, Buckingham.

Biggs JB, Tang C (2007) *Teaching for Quality Learning at University: What the Student Does,* 3rd edn. McGraw-Hill/Society for Research in Higher Education, Maidenhead.

Billett S (2004) Workplace participatory practices conceptualising workplaces as learning environments. *Journal of Workplace Learning,* 16, 312–324.

Bligh J, Brice J (2009) Further insights into the roles of the medical educator: the importance of scholarly management. *Academic Medicine,* 84, 1161–1165.

Bligh J, Prideaux D, Parsell G (2001) PRISMS: new educational strategies for medical education. *Medical Education,* 35, 520–521.

Bohmer R (2010) Leadership with a small 'l'. *BMJ,* 340, c483.

Boud D, Keogh R, Walker D (1989) *Reflection: Turning Experience into Learning.* Kogan Page, London.

Boursicot K, Etheridge L, Setna Z *et al.* (2011) Performance in assessment: consensus statements and recommendations from the Ottawa conference. *Medical Teacher,* 33, 370–383.

British Association for Counselling and Psychotherapy. Available at: www.bacp.co.uk/crs/Training/whatiscounselling.php (accessed August 2016).

Brookfield S (1993) Through the lens of learning: how the visceral experience of learning reframes teaching. In: BoudD, CohenR, WalkerD (eds). *Using Experience for Learning.* SHRE/Open University, Buckingham, pp. 19–21.

Buckley S, Coleman J, Davison I, *et al.* (2009) The educational effects of portfolios on undergraduate student learning. BEME guide 11. *Medical Teacher,* 31, 282–298.

Burford B, Ellis E, Williamson A, *et al.* (2015) Learning opportunities in 'student assistantships'. *The Clinical Teacher,* 12, 121–127.

Burgess A, McGregor D, Mellis C (2014) Medical students as peer tutors: a systematic review. *BMC Medical Education,* 14, 115.

Business Balls. Available at: www.businessballs.com (accessed August 2016).

Carnes M, Devine PG, Manwell LB, *et al.* (2015) The effect of an intervention to break the gender bias habit for faculty at one institution: a cluster randomized, controlled trial. *Academic Medicine,* 90, 221–230.

Carr PL, Gunn CM, Kaplan SA, *et al.* (2015) Inadequate progress for women in academic medicine: Findings from the national faculty study. *Journal of Women's Health,* 24, 190–199.

Caverzagie KJ, Cooney TG, Hemmer PA, Berkowitz L (2015) The development of entrustable professional activities for internal medicine residency training: A report from the education redesign committee of the alliance for academic internal medicine. *Academic Medicine,* 90, 479–484.

Centre for the Advancement of Interprofessional Education (CAIPE) (2002) Available at: http://caipe.org.uk/resources/defining-ipe (accessed Oct. 2016).

Charles G, Bainbridge L, Gilbert J (2010) The University of British Columbia model of IPE. *Journal of Interprofessional Care,* 24, 9–18.

Chew-Graham CA, Rogers A, Yassin N (2003) 'I wouldn't want it on my CV or their records': medical students' experiences of help-seeking for mental health problems. *Medical Education,* 37, 873–880.

Cleland JA, Knight LV, Rees CE, *et al.* (2008). Is it me or is it them? Factors that influence the passing of underperforming students. *Medical Education,* 42, 800–809.

Cleland JA, Nicholson S, Kelly N, Moffat M (2015) Taking context seriously: explaining widening access policy enactments in UK medical schools. *Medical Education,* 49, 25–35.

Clutterbuck D (2004) *Everyone Needs a Mentor: Fostering Talent in your Organisation.* CIPD Publishing.

Cook D (2014) When I say…validity. *Medical Education,* 48, 948–949.

Cooper N, Da Silva A, Powell S (2016) Teaching clinical reasoning. In: CooperN, FrainJ (eds) *ABC of Clinical Reasoning.* Wiley Blackwell, Chichester, pp. 44–50.

Crawley J (2005) *In at the Deep End – A Survival Guide for Teachers in Post Compulsory Education.* David Fulton, London.

Creative Commons. Available at: https://creativecommons.org (accessed August 2016).

Cresswell JW (2009) *Research Design. Qualitative, Quantitative and Mixed Methods Approaches.* Sage, London.

Croskerry P (2013) From mindless to mindful practice — cognitive bias and clinical decision making. *New England Journal of Medicine,* 368, 2445–2448.

Cruess RR, Johnston S, Cruess RL (2004) Profession: a working definition for medical educators. *Teaching and Learning in Medicine*, 16, 74–76.

Dauphinée D (1994) Determining the content of certification examinations. In: NewbleD, JollyB, WakefordR (eds) *The Certification and Recertification of Doctors: Issues in the Assessment of Clinical Competence*. Cambridge University Press, Cambridge, pp. 92–104.

Department of Health (2008) *Mental Health and Ill Health in Doctors*. Available at: http://webarchive.nationalarchives. gov.uk/+/www.dh.gov.uk/en/publicationsandstatistics/ publications/publicationspolicyandguidance/dh_083066 (accessed August 2016).

Dewey J (1933) *How We Think. A Restatement of the Relation of Reflective Thinking to the Educative Process* (revised edition). DC Heath, Boston.

Dreyfus HL, Dreyfus SE (1985) *Mind over Machine: the Power of Human Intuition and Expertise in the Era of the Computer*. Free Press, New York.

Driessen E, van der Vleuten C, Schuwirth L, *et al.* (2005) The use of qualitative research criteria for portfolio assessment as an alternative to reliability evaluation: a case study. *Medical Education*, 39, 214–220.

Duckworth A (2016) *Grit: The Power of Passion and Perseverance*. Simon and Schuster.

Dunning D, Heath C, Suls J (2004) Flawed self-assessment: implications for health, education, and the workplace. *Psychological Science in the Public Interest*, 5, 69–106.

Dyrbye LN, Thomas MR, Shanafelt TD (2006) Systematic review of depression, anxiety, and other indicators of psychological distress among US and Canadian medical students. *Academic Medicine*, 81, 354–373.

Dyrbye LN, West CP, Satele D, *et al.* (2014) Burnout among US medical students, residents, and early career physicians relative to the general US population. *Academic Medicine*, 89, 443–451.

Engeström Y (2007) Enriching the theory of expansive learning: Lessons from journeys toward co-configuration. *Mind Culture and Activity*, 14, 23–39.

EppichWJ, O'ConnorL, AdlerM (2013) Providing effective simulation activities. In: ForrestK, McKimmJ, EdgarS (eds) *Essential Simulation in Clinical Education*. Wiley Blackwell, Chichester, pp. 213–234.

Equality Challenge Unit (ECU) (2013) *Unconscious Bias Training Materials*. Available at: www.ecu.ac.uk/wp-content/ uploads/2014/07/unconscious-bias-and-higher-education.pdf (accessed Oct. 2016).

Ericsson A, Krampe R, Tesch-Romer C (1993) The role of deliberate practice in the acquisition of expert performance. *Psychological Review*, 100, 363–406.

Ericsson KA (2004) Deliberate practice and the acquisition and maintenance of expert performance in medicine and related domains. *Academic Medicine*, 79 (Suppl), S70–S81.

European Commission. *Education and Training, the Bologna Process*. Available at: http://ec.europa.eu/dgs/education_ culture/repository/education/library/publications/2015/ bologna-process-brochure_en.pdf (accessed Oct. 2015).

Eva KW, Armson H, Holmboe E, *et al.* (2012) Factors influencing responsiveness to feedback: on the interplay between fear, confidence and reasoning processes. *Advances in Health Sciences Education*, 17, 15–26.

Eva KW, Macala C (2014) Multiple mini-interview test characteristics: 'tis better to ask candidates to recall than to imagine. *Medical Education*, 48, 604–613.

Eve R (2003) *PUNs and DENs. Discovering Learning Needs in General Practice*. Radcliffe Medical Press, Abingdon.

Fincher RM, Work J (2006) Perspectives on the scholarship of teaching. *Medical Education*, 40, 293–295.

Flexner A (1910) *Medical Education in the United States and Canada: A Report to the Carnegie Foundation for the Advancement of Teaching*. Carnegie Foundation for the Advancement of Teaching, New York.

ForrestK, McKimmJ, EdgarS (eds) (2013) *Essential Simulation in Clinical Education*. Wiley Blackwell.

FrankJR, SnellL, SherbinoJ (eds) (2015) *The Draft CanMEDS 2015 Physician Competency Framework*, Series IV. Royal College of Physicians and Surgeons of Canada, Ottawa.

Frenk J, Chen L, Bhutta ZA, *et al.* (2010) Health professionals for a new century: transforming education to strengthen health systems in an interdependent world. *Lancet*, 376, 1923–1958.

Garvey B, Garrett-Harris R (2005) *The Benefits of Mentoring: A Literature Review, A Report for East Mentors Forum*. Coaching and Mentoring Research Unit, Sheffield Hallam University, Sheffield.

General Medical Council (GMC) (1993) *Tomorrow's Doctors*. GMC, London.

General Medical Council (GMC) (2009) *Tomorrow's Doctors*. GMC, London.

General Medical Council (GMC) (2013a) *Doctors' use of social media*. Available at: www.gmc-uk.org/static/documents/ content/Doctors_use_of_social_media.pdf (accessed August 2016).

General Medical Council (GMC) (2013b) *Good Medical Practice*. GMC, London.

General Practitioner Education and Training (GPET) (2013) *A Framework for Vertical Integration in GP Education and Training*. General Practice Education and Training Ltd, Canberra.

Gibbs G (1988) *Learning by Doing: A Guide to Teaching and Learning Methods*. Oxford Further Education Unit, Oxford.

Gleeson F (1997) AMEE Medical Education Guide No. 9. Assessment of clinical competence using the Objective Structured Long Examination Record (OSLER). *Medical Teacher*, 19, 7–14.

Global Consensus on Social Accountability of Medical Schools. Available at: http://healthsocialaccountability.org (accessed July 2016).

Goldie J (2013) Assessment of professionalism: A consolidation of current thinking. *Medical Teacher*, 35, e952–e956.

Goleman D (2000) *Leadership that Gets Results*. Available at: www.defence.gov.au/ADC/Docs/CDLE/CDLE_120329_ Goleman2000LeadershipthatGetsResults.pdf (accessed Oct. 2016).

Gordon J (2003) ABC of learning and teaching in medicine: one to one teaching and feedback. *BMJ*, 326 (7388), 543–545.

Grant A (2013) *Reflection and Medical Students' Learning: an In-Depth Study Combining Qualitative and Qualitative Methodologies*. Lambert Academic Publishing, Saarbrücken, Germany.

Grant J (2014) Principles of curriculum design. In: SwanwickT (ed) *Understanding Medical Education: Evidence, Theory and Practice*, 2nd edn. Wiley Blackwell/ASME, Chichester, pp. 31–46.

Greenwood J (1998) The role of reflection in single and double loop learning. *Journal of Advanced Learning*, 27, 1048–1053.

Gross AG, Walzer AE (2000) *Rereading Aristotle's Rhetoric*. Southern Illinois University Press, Carbondale, IL, USA.

Haider S, Johnson N, Thistlethwaite JE, *et al.* (2015) WATCH: Warwick Assessment insTrument for Clinical teacHing: Development and testing. *Medical Teacher*, 37, 289–295.

Harden R (2006) International medical education and future directions: A global perspective. *Academic Medicine*, 81, S22–S29.

Harden R, Gleeson FA (1979) Assessment of clinical competence using an objective structured clinical examination (OSCE). *Medical Education*, 13, 39–54.

Harden R, Stevenson W, Downie WW, Wilson G (1975) Assessment of clinical competence using objective structured clinical examination. *BMJ*, 5995, 447–451.

Harden RM (2007) Outcome-based education–the ostrich, the peacock and the beaver. *Medical Teacher*, 29, 666–671.

Harden RM, Sowden S, Dunn WR (1984) Educational strategies in curriculum development: the SPICES model. *Medical Education*, 18, 284–297.

Hays RB, Lawson M, Gray C (2011) Problems presented by medical students seeking support: A possible intervention framework. *Medical Teacher*, 33, 161–164.

Health Foundation (2011) *Can Patients be Teachers?* Health Foundation, London.

Health Research Authority (2013) *Defining Research*. NHS. Available at: www.hra.nhs.uk/documents/2016/06/defining-research.pdf.

Heron J (1986) *Six Category Intervention Analysis*. Human Potential Research Project, University of Guildford, Surrey.

Hesketh EA, Laidlaw JM (2002) Developing the teaching instinct: feedback. *Medical Teacher*, 24, 245–248.

Hicks PJ, Cox SM, Espey EL, *et al.* (2005) To the point: medical education reviews – dealing with student difficulties in the clinical setting. *American Journal of Obstetrics and Gynaecology*, 193, 1915–1922.

Higher Education Academy (2015) *Embedding Equality and Diversity into the Curriculum*: *A Practitioners' Guide*. Available at: https://www.heacademy.ac.uk/sites/default/files/resources/eedc_education_online.pdf (accessed May 2016).

Hilton SR, Slotnick HB (2005) Proto-professionalism: how professionalisation occurs across the continuum of medical education. *Medical Education*, 39, 58–65.

HodgesBD, LingardL (2012) (eds) *The question of Competence: Reconsidering Medical Education in the 21st Century*. Cornell University Press, Ithaca, NY.

Howe A, Anderson J (2003) Involving patients in medical education. *BMJ*, 327(7410), 326–328.

Hurtubise L, Hall E, Sheridan L, Han H (2015) The flipped classroom in medical education: engaging students to build competency. *Journal of Medical Education and Curricular Development*, 2, 35–43.

Hussey T, Smith P (2003) The uses of learning outcomes. *Teaching in Higher Education*, 8, 357–368.

Institute for International Medical Education (IIME) Available at: www.iime.org (accessed May 2015).

Institute for International Medical Education (IIME) (2016) *Glossary of Medical Terms*. Available at: www.iime.org/glossary.htm#M (assessed Oct. 2016).

Issenberg SB, McGaghie WC, Petrusa ER, *et al.* (2005) Features and uses of high fidelity medical simulations that lead to effective learning: a BEME systematic review. *Medical Teacher*, 27, 10–28.

Jacques D (2010) Teaching small groups. In: CantillonP, WoodD (eds) *ABC of Learning and Teaching in Medicine*, 2nd edn. Wiley Blackwell/BMJ Books, Chichester, pp. 23–28.

Jisc (2010) *Open Educational Resources* (OERs). Available at: https://www.jisc.ac.uk/guides/open-educational-resources (accessed April 2016).

Kahneman D (2012) *Thinking, Fast and Slow*. Penguin, London.

Kaufman DM, Mann KV (2014) Teaching and learning in medical education: how theory can inform practice. In: SwanwickT (ed) *Understanding Medical Education: Evidence, Theory and Practice*. ASME/Wiley Blackwell, Chichester, pp. 7–30.

Kelley RE (1988) In praise of followers. *Harvard Business Review*, 66, 142–148.

Kilminster SM, Jolly BC (2000) Effective supervision in clinical practice settings: a literature review. *Medical Education*, 34, 827–840.

Kirkpatrick D, Kirkpatrick J (2006) *Evaluating Training Programs: The Four Level Model*. Berrett-Koehler, San Francisco.

Kjeldstadli K, Tyssen R, Finset A, *et al.* (2006) Life satisfaction and resilience in medical school–a six-year longitudinal, nationwide and comparative study. *BMC Medical Education*, 6, 48.

Kneebone R, Arora S, King D, *et al.* (2010) Distributed simulation – accessible immersive training. *Medical Teacher*, 32, 65–70.

Kogan JR, Holmboe ES, Hauer KE (2009) Tools for direct observation and assessment of clinical skills of medical trainees: a systematic review. *JAMA*, 302, 1316–1326.

Kolb DA (1984) *Experiential Learning: Experience as the Source of Learning and Development*. Prentice Hall, Englewood-Cliffs, NJ.

Kolb DA, Fry RE (1975) Towards an applied theory of experiential learning. In: CooperCL (ed) *Theories of Group Processes*. Wiley, London, pp. 33–58.

Lake F, Ryan G (2004) Teaching on the run tip no 4: teaching with patients. *Medical Journal of Australia*, 181, 158–159.

Lave J, Wenger E (1991) *Situated Learning: Legitimate Peripheral Participation*. Cambridge University Press, Cambridge.

Lave J, Wenger E (1999) *Legitimate Peripheral Participation. Learners, Learning and Assessment*. Open University, London, pp. 83–89.

Lee A, Steketee C, Rogers G, Moran, M (2013) Towards a theoretical framework for curriculum development in health professional education. *Focus on Health Professional Education*, 14, 70–83.

Leonard M, Graham S, Bonacum D (2004) The human factor: the critical importance of effective teamwork and communication in providing safe care. *Quality and Safety in Health Care*, 13 (Suppl.1), i85–90.

Lincoln YS, Lynham SA, Guba EG (2011) Paradigmatic controversies, contradictions, and emerging confluences, revisited. *Sage Handbook of Qualitative Research*, 4, 97–128.

Lueddeke GR (2012) *Transforming Medical Education for the 21st Century*. Radcliffe Publishing Ltd, London.

Luft J, Ingham H (1955) *The Johari Window, a Graphic Model of Interpersonal Awareness*. Proceedings of the Western Training Laboratory in Group Development, University of California, Los Angeles.

Lyon P (2004) A model of teaching and learning in the operating theatre. *Medical Education*, 38, 1278–1287.

Mann KV, Dornan T, Teunissen PW (2011) Perspectives on learning. In: DornanT, MannK, ScherpbierA, SpencerJ (eds)

Medical Education: Theory and Practice. Churchill Livingstone/Elsevier, Edinburgh, pp. 17–38.

Marton GE, McCullough B, Ramanan CJ (2015) A review of teaching skills development programmes for medical students. *Medical Education*, 49, 149–160.

McGaghie WC, Issenberg SB, Petrusa ER, *et al.* (2010) A critical review of simulation-based medical education research: 2003–2009. *Medical Education*, 44, 50–63.

McKimm J (2008) *Involving Patients in Clinical Teaching.* London Deanery, London. Available at: http://www.faculty.londondeanery.ac.uk/e-learning/involving-patients-in-health-professions-education (accessed Oct. 2016).

McKimm J (2009) *Assessing Educational Needs.* Multiprofessional Faculty Development. NHS Health Education England. Available at: www.faculty.londondeanery.ac.uk/e-learning/assessing-educational-needs (accessed Oct. 2016).

McKimm J, Morris C (2014) *Small Group Teaching NHS Health Education Central, East, North West and South London.* Available at: www.faculty.londondeanery.ac.uk/e-learning/small-group-teaching (accessed August 2016).

McKimm J, Newton PH, Campbell J, *et al.* (2013) *Medical Education: A Review of International Trends and Current Approaches in Pacific Island Countries.* Human Resources for Health Knowledge Hub, Sydney, Australia. Available at: www.hrhhub.unsw.edu.au (accessed May 2015).

McKimm J, O'Sullivan H (2016) When I say … Leadership. *Medical Education*, 50, 896–897.

McKimm J, Vogan C, Jones P (2016) *Leadership in 3s.* Workshop presentation at ASME Annual Scientific Meeting, 6 July 2016, Belfast.

McKimm J, Wilkinson T (2015) "Doctors on the move": Exploring professionalism in the light of cultural transitions. *Medical Teacher*, 37, 837–843.

McLean M, McKimm J, Major S (2014) Medical educators working abroad: A pilot study of educators' experiences in the Middle East. *Medical Teacher*, 36, 757–764.

McManus IC, Woolf K, Dacre J, *et al.* (2013) The academic backbone: longitudinal continuities in educational achievement from secondary school and medical school to MRCP (UK) and the specialist register in UK medical students and doctors. *BMC Medicine*, 11, 1.

Medical Schools' Council and General Medical Council (2015). *Supporting Medical Students with Mental Health Conditions.* MSC and GMC (published July 2013; updated July 2015). Available at: www.gmc-uk.org/Supporting_students_with_mental_health_conditions_0816.pdf_53047904.pdf (accessed Oct. 2016).

Mehrabian A (1971) *Silent Messages*, 1st edn. Wadsworth, Belmont, CA.

Merriam SB, Caffarella RS, Baumgartner LM (2007) *Learning in Adulthood: a Comprehensive Guide.* Jossey-Bass, San Francisco.

Mezirow J (1991) *Transformative Dimensions of Adult Learning.* Jossey-Bass, San Francisco.

Miller A, Archer J (2010) Impact of workplace based assessment on doctors' education and performance: a systematic review. *BMJ*, 341, c5064.

Miller GE (1990) The assessment of clinical skills/competence/performance. *Academic Medicine*, 65 (Suppl), S63–S67.

Miller HL (1927) *Creative Learning and Teaching.* HathiTrust, Charles Scribner's Sons, New York.

Monrouxe, LV, Rees, CE (2009) Picking up the gauntlet: constructing medical education as a social science. *Medical Education*, 43, 196–198.

Moon J (1999) *Reflection in Learning and Professional Development.* Kogan Page, London.

Moon J (2004) *A Handbook of Reflective and Experiential Learning: Theory and Practice.* Routledge, London.

Morris C, Blaney D (2014) Work-based learning. In: Swanwick T (ed) *Understanding Medical Education: Evidence, Theory and Practice.* ASME/Wiley Blackwell, Chichester, pp. 97–110.

Neher JO, Gordon KA, Meyer B (1992) A five-step 'microskills' method of clinical teaching. *Journal of the American Board of Family Practice*, 5, 419–424.

Nestel D, Bearman M (2015) *Simulated Patient Methodology. Theory, Evidence and Practice.* Wiley Blackwell, Chichester.

Nicholson S, Cleland J (2015) Reframing research on widening participation in medical education: using theory to inform practice. *Researching Medical Education*, 18, 231.

Nickson CP, Cadogan MD (2014) Free open access medical education (FOAM) for the emergency physician. *Emergency Medicine Australasia*, 26, 76–83.

Norcini JJ, Blank LL, Duffy FD, Fortna GS (2003) The mini-CES: a method for assessing clinical skills. *Annals of Internal Medicine*, 138, 476–481.

Northouse, PG (2010) *Leadership Theory and Practice.* Sage, London.

O'Brien L (2015) Problem-based learning: best evidence in health professional learning. In: Brown T, Williams B (eds) *Evidence-Based Education in the Health Professions.* Radcliffe Publishing Ltd, London, pp. 288–300.

Orrell J (2006) Good practice report: Work-integrated learning. *Australian Learning and Teaching Council*, Surry Hills, NSW.

Østergaard D, Rosenberg J (2013) The evidence: what works, why and how? In: Forrest K, McKimm J, Edgar S (eds) *Essential Simulation in Clinical Education.* Wiley Blackwell, Chichester, pp. 26–42.

Oxford English Dictionary (2016) Available at: www.oed.com/view/Entry/152054?redirectedFrom=professionalism#eid (accessed Oct. 2016).

Patterson F, Rowett E, Hale R, *et al.* (2016) The predictive validity of a situational judgement test and multiple-mini interview for entry into postgraduate training in Australia. *BMC Medical Education*, 16, 1.

Patton MQ (2008) *Utilization-Focused Evaluation*, 4th edn. Sage, Los Angeles.

Pawson R, Tilley N (1997) *Realistic Evaluation.* Sage, London.

Pearsall J (2002) *Concise Oxford English Dictionary*, 10th revised edn. Oxford University Press, UK.

Pendleton D, Schofield T, Tate P and Havelock P (1984) *The Consultation: an Approach to Learning and Teaching.* Oxford University Press, Oxford.

Petrie N (2014) *Vertical Leadership Development. Part 1 Developing Leaders for a Complex World.* Center for Creative Leadership. Available at: http://www.ccl.org/leadership/pdf/research/VerticalLeadersPart1.Pdf (accessed Oct. 2016).

Ramsden P (1992) *Learning to Teach in Higher Education.* Routledge, London.

Rees C, Monrouxe L, McDonald L (2013) Narrative, emotion and action: analysing 'most memorable' professionalism dilemmas. *Medical Education*, 47, 80–96.

Regan-Smith M, Hirschmann K, Iobst W (2007) Direct observation of faculty with feedback: an effective means of improving patient-centered and learner-centered teaching skills. *Teaching and Learning in Medicine*, 19, 278–286.

Rethans J-J, Norcini JJ, Baron-Maldonado M, *et al.* (2002) The relationship between competence and performance: implications for assessing practice performance. *Medical Education*, 36, 901–909.

Rethans J-J, Sturmans F, Drop R, *et al.* (1991) Does competence of general practitioners predict their performance? Comparison between examination setting and actual practice. *BMJ*, 303, 1377–1380.

Riley RH, Grauze AM, Chinnery C, *et al.* (2003) Three years of 'CASMS": the world's busiest medical simulation centre. *Medical Journal of Australia*, 179, 626–630.

Ross MT, Cameron H (2007) Peer assisted learning: a planning and implementation framework. AMEE Guide No. 30. *Medical Teacher*, 29, 527–545.

Rossi P, Lipsey MW, Freeman HE (2004) *Evaluation: a Systematic Approach*, 7th ed. Sage, Thousand Oaks.

Royal College of Physicians and Surgeons of Canada (CANMEDS) (2015) Available at: www.royalcollege.ca/rcsite/canmeds-e (accessed Oct. 2016).

Rudolph JW, Simon R, Dufresne RL, Raemer DB (2006) There's no such thing as 'nonjudgemental debriefing': a theory and model for debriefing with good judgement. *Simulation in Healthcare*, 2, 115–125.

Schmidt RA (1991) Frequent augmented feedback can degrade learning: Evidence and interpretations. In: StelmachGE, RequinJ (eds) *Tutorials in Motor Neuroscience*. Kluwer, Dordrecht, pp. 59–76.

Schön DA (1983). *The Reflective Practitioner: How Professionals Think in Action*. Basic Books, New York.

Schön, DA (1987) *Educating the Reflective Practitioner: Toward a New Design for Teaching and Learning in the Professions*. Jossey-Bass, San Francisco.

Scully M, Rowe M (2009) Bystander training within organizations. *Journal of the International Ombudsman Association*, 2, 1–9.

Seagraves L, Boyd A (1996) *Supporting Learners in the Workplace: Guidelines for Learning Advisers in Small and Medium-Sized Companies*. University of Stirling, Stirling.

Secomb J (2008) A systematic review of peer teaching and learning in clinical education. *Journal of Clinical Nursing*, 17, 703–716.

Silverman J, Kurtz S, Draper J (2005) *Skills for Communicating with Patients*. Radcliffe Medical Press, Abingdon.

Silverman JD, Kurtz SM, Draper J (1996) The Calgary Cambridge approach to communication skills teaching 1: Agenda-led, outcome-based analysis of the consultation. *Education for General Practice*, 4, 288–299.

Simmons B, Egan-Lee E, Wagner SJ, *et al.* (2011) Assessment of interprofessional learning: The design of an interprofessional objective structured clinical examination (iOSCE) approach. *Journal of Interprofessional Care*, 25, 73–74.

Snadden D, Thomas ML (1998) The use of portfolio learning in medical education. *Medical Teacher*, 20, 192–199.

Southgate L, Grant J (2004) *Principles for an Assessment System for Postgraduate Training*. Postgraduate Medical Education and Training Board (PMETB), London.

Sox H, Higgins MC, Owens DK (2013) *Medical Decision Making*, 2nd edn. Wiley-Blackwell, Chichester.

Spencer J, Blackmore D, Heard S, *et al.* (2000) Patient-oriented learning: A review of the role of the patient in the education of medical students. *Medical Education*, 34, 851–857.

Spencer J, McKimm J (2014) Patient involvement in medical education. In: SwanwickT (ed) *Understanding Medical Education: Evidence, Theory and Practice*, 2nd edn. ASME/Wiley Blackwell, Chichester, pp. 227–240.

Spencer JA (2010) Learning and teaching in the clinical environment. In: Cantillon, P, Wood, D (eds) *ABC of Learning and Teaching*, 2nd edn. Wiley BMJ Books, Chichester, pp. 33–37.

Srinivasan M, Wilkes M, Stevenson F, *et al.* (2007) Comparing problem-based learning with case-based learning: effects of a major curricular shift at two institutions. *Academic Medicine*, 82, 74–82.

Stewart M, Brown JB, Weston WW, *et al.* (1995) *Patient-Centered Medicine. Transforming the Clinical Method*. Sage, California.

Stuart J, Rutherford R (1978) Medical student concentration during lectures. *Lancet*, 2, 514–516.

Sturdy S (2007) Scientific method for medical practitioners: the case method of teaching pathology in early twentieth-century Edinburgh. *Bulletin of the History of Medicine*, 81, 760–792.

Swanwick T (2005) Informal learning in postgraduate medical education: from cognitivism to 'culturalism'. *Medical Education*, 39, 859–865.

Swanwick T (2014) Understanding medical education. In: SwanwickT (ed) *Understanding Medical Education: Evidence, Theory and Practice*, 2nd edn. Wiley Blackwell/ASME, Chichester, pp. 3–6.

SwanwickT (ed) *Understanding Medical Education: Evidence, Theory and Practice*, 2nd edn. Wiley Blackwell/ASME, Chichester.

Swanwick T, McKimm J (2014). Faculty development for leadership and management. In: SteinertY (ed) *Faculty Development in the Health Professions: A Focus on Research and Practice*. Dordrecht: Springer, pp. 53–78.

Symonds I, Cullen L, Fraser D (2003) Evaluation of a formative interprofessional team objective structured clinical examination (ITOSCE): A method of shared learning in maternity education. *Medical Teacher*, 25, 38–41.

Tan N, Sutton A, Dornan T (2011) Morality and philosophy of medicine and education. In: DornanT, MannK, ScherpbierA, SpencerJ (eds) *Medical Education: Theory and Practice*. Churchill Livingstone Elsevier, Edinburgh, pp. 3–16.

Tang J, Tun JK, Kneebone RL, Bello F (2013) Distributed simulation. In: ForrestK, McKimmJ, EdgarS (eds) *Essential Simulation in Clinical Education*. Wiley Blackwell, Chichester, pp. 196–212.

ten Cate O, Durning S (2007a) Dimensions and psychology of peer teaching in medical education. *Medical Teacher*, 29, 546–52.

ten Cate O, Durning S (2007b) Peer teaching in medical education: twelve reasons to move from theory to practice. *Medical Teacher*, 29, 591–599.

Tew J, Gell, C, Foster S (2004) *Learning from Experience. Involving Service Users and Carers in Mental Health Education and Training*. Higher Education Academy/NIMHE/Trent Workforce Development Confederation, Nottingham.

Thistlethwaite J (2015a) When I say…realism. *Medical Education*, 49, 459–460.

Thistlethwaite JE (2015b) Assessment of interprofessional teamwork – an international perspective. In: FormanD, JonesM, ThistlethwaiteJE (eds) *Leadership and Collaboration*. Palgrave, Basingstoke, pp. 35–152.

Thistlethwaite JE (2015c) Case-based learning: application and evidence in health professional education. In: BrownT, WilliamsB (eds) *Evidence-based Education in the Health Professions*. Radcliffe Publishing Ltd, London, pp. 301–312.

Thistlethwaite JE, Bartle E, Chong AL *et al.* (2013) A review of longitudinal community and hospital placements in medical education: BEME Guide No. 26. *Medical Teacher*, 35, e1340–1364.

Thistlethwaite JE, Davies H, Dornan T, *et al.* (2012a) What is evidence? Reflections on the AMEE symposium, Vienna, August 2011. *Medical Teacher*, 34, 453–457.

Thistlethwaite JE, Davies D, Ekeocha S, *et al.* (2012b) The effectiveness of case-based learning in health professional education: A BEME systematic review. *Medical Teacher*, 34, e421–e444.

Thistlethwaite JE, Moran M (2010) Learning outcomes for IPE: literature review and synthesis. *Journal of Interprofessional Care*, 24, 503–513.

Thistlethwaite JE, Moran M, Kumar K, *et al.* (2015) An exploratory review of pre-qualification interprofessional education evaluations. *Journal of Interprofessional Care*, 29, 292–297.

Thistlethwaite JE, Morris P (2006) *Patient-Doctor Consultations in Primary Care: Theory and Practice*. Royal College of General Practitioners, London.

Till A, Pettifer G, O'Sullivan H, McKimm J (2014) Developing and harnessing the leadership potential of doctors in training, *British Journal of Hospital Medicine*, 75 281–285.

Tochel C, Haig A, Hesketh A, *et al.* (2009) The effectiveness of portfolios for post-graduate assessment and education. BEME guide 12. *Medical Teacher*, 31, 299–318.

Topping KJ (1996) The effectiveness of peer tutoring in further and higher education: a typology and review of the literature. *Higher Education*, 32, 321–345.

Towle A, Bainbridge L, Godolphin W, *et al.* (2010) Active patient involvement in the education of health professionals. *Medical Education*, 44, 64–74.

Towle A, Godolphin W (2015) Patients as teachers: promoting their authentic and autonomous voices. *The Clinical Teacher*, 12, 149–154.

Trochim WMK (2006) Research methods knowledge base. Available at: www.socialresearchmethods.net/kb/positvsm.php (accessed August 2016).

Trowbridge RL, Graber ML (2015) Clinical reasoning and diagnostic error. In: TrowbridgeRL, RencicJJ, DurningSJ (eds) *Teaching Clinical Reasoning*. American College of Physicians, Philadelphia.

Tsui ABM, Lopez-Real F, Edwards G (2009) Sociocultural perspectives of learning. In: TsuiABM, EdwardsG, Lopez-RealF (eds) *Learning in School-University Partnership, Sociocultural Perspectives*. Routledge, New York, pp. 25–44.

Tuckett D, Boulton M, Olson C, Williams A (1985) *Meetings Between Experts: an Approach to Sharing Ideas in Medical Consultations*. Tavistock Publications, London.

Van der Ridder JMM, Stokking KM, McGaghie WC, ten Cate OTJ (2008). What is feedback in clinical education? *Medical Education*, 42, 189–197.

Van der Vleuten C (1996) The assessment of professional competence: developments, research and practical implications. *Advances in Health Sciences Education*, 1, 41–67.

Van der Vleuten C, Schuwirth L, Driessen EW, *et al.* (2012) A model for programmatic assessment fit for purpose. *Medical Teacher*, 34, 205–214.

Vogan CL, McKimm J, Da Silva AL, Grant A (2014a) Twelve tips for providing effective student support in undergraduate medical education. *Medical Teacher*, 36, 480–485.

Vogan CL, McKimm J, Jones PK, *et al.* (2014b) The Swansea 6D model: a tool to help provide appropriate student support. Poster presentation, *ASME Annual Scientific Meeting*, Brighton, UK (July 16–18).

Vogan CL, McKimm J, Murtagh J, *et al.* (2013) The Web of Support: Providing Effective Support to Medical Students on Clinical Placement. Poster presentation, *17th Annual IAMSE Meeting*, St. Andrews, Scotland, UK (June 8 – 11, 2013).

von Fragstein M, Silverman J, Cushing A, *et al.* (2008) UK consensus statement on the content of communication curricula in undergraduate medical education. *Medical Education*, 42, 1100–1107.

Vygotsky L (1978) *Mind in Society: the Development of Higher Psychological Processes*. Harvard University Press, Cambridge, MA.

Walsh K (2005) The rules. *British Medical Journal*, 331, 574.

Whitmore J (2009) *Coaching for Performance*, 4th edn. Nicholas Brealey Publishing, London.

Wilkinson TJ, Harris P (2002) The transition out of medical school–a qualitative study of descriptions of borderline trainee interns. *Medical Education*, 36, 466–471.

Wong G, Greenhalgh T, Westhorp G, Pawson R (2012) Realist methods in medical education research: what are they and what can they contribute? *Medical Education*, 46, 89–96.

World Federation of Medical Education (WFME) (2016) Available at: http://wfme.org (accessed Oct. 2016).

World Health Organization (WHO) (2010a) *Framework for Action on Interprofessional Education and Collaborative Practice*. WHO, Geneva.

World Health Organization (WHO) (2013) *Transforming and Scaling Up Health Professionals' Education and Training*. WHO, Geneva.

Yardley S, Dornan T (2012) Kirkpatrick's levels and education 'evidence'. *Medical Education*, 46, 97–106.

Yates J (2011) Development of a 'toolkit' to identify medical students at risk of failure to thrive on the course: an exploratory retrospective case study. *BMC Medical Education*, 11, 95.

Yepes-Roi M, Varpio L, Duboyce R, *et al.* (2015) *Failure to Fail Underperforming Trainees in Health Professions: A BEME Systematic Review of the Barriers Inhibiting Educators*. Available at: http://bemecollaboration.org/Reviews+In+Progress/Failure+to+Fail// (accessed August 2016).

Index

Medical Education at a Glance, First Edition. Edited by Judy McKimm, Kirsty Forrest and Jill Thistlethwaite © 2017 John Wiley & Sons, Ltd. Published 2017 by John Wiley & Sons, Ltd.